Praise for *Second Spring*

'What a tremendous contribution Kate has made to the conversation on menopause and to women at this stage of life. If you want to do menopause differently than what our society tells us it must be, if you feel an inkling to take back menopause on your terms, then get this book. I can think of dozens of women I want to send this book to!'
Karen Brody, Founder, Daring to Rest and author of *Daring to Rest: Reclaim Your Power with Yoga Nidra Rest Meditation.*

'With the warm hug of a kind friend, on point humour and the ease of well-honed expertise Kate Codrington has written an essential companion for women from pre perimenopause through to post-menopause. Much as I would have loved to have had this book as my own companion when this all began for me 20 years ago, but I am so grateful for Kate's insights and tips now, and to finally have a book I can wholeheartedly recommend on this ubiquitous, yet seriously ignored, underfunded and disparaged experience.
**Jane Bennett, menstrual educator and author,
founder Chalice Foundation.**

'Second Spring reads like the voice of a dear and wise friend sharing her hard-earned wisdom and secrets. In cultures focused on youth, menopause can be a lonely time. Kate Codrington has sourced a wealth of seasoned guidance to navigate and celebrate the mind body and spirit aspects of the menopausal journey.'
Tami Lynn Kent, author of *Wild Feminine, Wild Creative & Mothering from Your Center.*

'This book is chock full of ideas about how to not simply get through menopause, but also how to grow through menopause. It rides the fine line between acknowledging the awful truths that are part of this change while at the same time holding out hope for what comes next. There is no one-size-fits-all map for menopause, and this book offers a wide variety of suggestions and resources to choose from.
Jane Cawthorne, Co-Editor, *Writing Menopause: An Anthology of Fiction, Poetry and Creative Non-Fiction.*

'This is a wonderful book to accompany you through menopause. Wise, irreverent and above all kind. It will help you navigate the seeming madness and suffering that too many experience. Instead of feeling it's the end, you might just discover yourself, and that can only spell freedom.
Alexandra Pope, co-author of *Wild Power: discover the magic of menstrual cycle and awaken the feminine path to power.*

Second Spring

The Self-Care Guide to Menopause

Kate Codrington

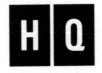

ONE PLACE. MANY STORIES

HQ
An imprint of HarperCollins*Publishers* Ltd
1 London Bridge Street
London SE1 9GF

www.harpercollins.co.uk

HarperCollins *Publishers*
1st Floor, Watermarque Building, Ringsend Road, Dublin 4, Ireland

1
First published in Great Britain by
HQ, an imprint of HarperCollins*Publishers* Ltd 2021

ISBN: 978-0-00-846975-7

MIX
Paper from
responsible sources
FSC
www.fsc.org
FSC™ C007454

This book is produced from independently certified FSC™ paper
to ensure responsible forest management.

For more information visit: www.harpercollins.co.uk/green

This book is set in 11/14 pt. pt. Bell MT by Type-it AS. Norway

Printed and Bound in the UK using 100% Renewable Electricity at
CPI Group (UK) Ltd, Croydon, CR0 4YY

For Bella

Contents

Foreword

Menopause is transformative. It's a magnificent challenge in the cycles of our lives, an opportunity to evolve and grow. Menopause is a loud call to re-evaluate who we think we are, and to become our true selves with authenticity and grace. It is the immense power of cyclical wisdom, turning the light of middle-aged wisdom in upon our own selves. It is time to illuminate our shadows, to reclaim, re-make and reconnect to our essential nature.

When I first met a perimenopausal Kate Codrington, she announced to me her intention to have a 'kick-ass menopause!'. And over the years I watched in admiration as Kate approached her own menopause with a full and openhearted commitment to the process. She did indeed navigate a kick-ass menopause: creative, hilarious, well rested, honest and profound. The wisdom she shares in this companion to the menopausal journey is rooted not just in her own experience, but in the lives of the many women for whom she has become a guide and inspiration. This is not an ordinary kind of guidebook. It doesn't tell you what to do – it is more of a generous and supportive companion who makes suggestions and encourages you to listen to your own intuition. Kate's writing is the ideal companion for the journey of menopause. And believe me, the menopausal journey is not a journey anyone should make alone. It is a journey that needs courage, and encouragement, the companionship of fellow travellers on the path . . .

For the energy of menopause is a vital force for freedom, working through the evolution of soul, heart and mind to transform every level of our being, from the physical to the emotional, from the sexual to the intuitive, from the mind to the psyche to the soul. Stepping through the door of menopause we step into our full power, we step up into the capacity to see clearly, and we step forwards to show others the way to freedom.

So why is it so feared and so reviled?

Because freedom is disruptive! Our mainstream culture fears the disruptive power of women's freedom, and does everything in its power to make sure we cannot even see this door to liberation. Our cultural prejudice against ageing and our youth-obsessed media promote such deep shame, disgust, and embarrassment at the bodies of menopausal women that millions of us simply put down our heads and walk on past the door marked 'Menopausal Transformation'. We are too repulsed by our own ageing to notice the gifts it can bring. We fear the existence of menopause, and deny our own cyclical wisdom.

Why? Because almost everything about our society is geared to disconnect us from any kind of cyclical wisdom. The lords of profit to whom we are enslaved by the corporations for whom many of us work do not want us to access our own wisdom. The rhythmic cycles of menstruation, pregnancies, and menopause disrupt the structures of capitalist economies, and so we are taught to deny that we are cyclical beings, to behave like men, to denigrate our most intimate and precious intuitions and insights. And since our mutable and cyclical nature cannot be entirely eradicated, we are taught to be ashamed of it, ashamed of our blood, ashamed of our wrinkles, ashamed of our white hairs, ashamed of our intuition; menstrual shame leads to sexual shame, which leads to profound disconnection and disempowerment, all of which leads to menopausal suffering at every level of being.

And yet, despite all the bad press, and the attempts to distract, delude, and disempower us, we still find ourselves stumbling towards freedom. We are in the company of an extraordinary demographic – for there are more menopausal women alive on this planet now than at any previous point in human history. And so we can be guided by the voices of those who are not ashamed, of those who celebrate the magnificence of this challenge to grow down into ourselves. The brave voices of women such as Kate, who have travelled through menopause with dignity, self-awareness, and humour, these voices call us to honour our own journeys and call us to honour ourselves.

The process of menopause, through which I am travelling still, is the most powerful initiation of my life. And it is the voices of my sisters that have helped me to recognize this. At 54, I was only part way through my first year with no bleeds, when Kate sent me a draft of this book. I was uplifted and inspired by what she shares in these pages, and so I agreed to write this foreword. But it took me months and months, because I was journeying through the terrain of menopause and everything looked different, and deadlines somehow didn't mean the same to me anymore. There was always something else calling my attention, and my journey into transformative surrender was deep and complete. As the days since my last period turned into three digit numbers, I launched a campaign to eradicate the abuse of women in yoga. As the days since my last period reached over 200, I followed Kate's advice about 'taking a menopausal gap year' and I retreated to the far west of Ireland. I hid out on the wild coast of Clare to work on finishing a book I have been writing for the past seven years. The process of writing this book, which I still have not finished, is the calendar of my menopause, a journey still incomplete. I am still a traveller on the menopausal journey, as I have been for the past seven years.

The territory of menopause is vast, and each one of us has her own unique journey to make. Kate has many wise counsels and hilarious observations to make about the process of travelling in this terrain. She is a generous and curious companion, open to all that can arise. The tips she offers and the stages she describes are not set in stone, and each one of us can take wisdom from the patterns Kate describes. We can also be open to the surprises that unfold along the path. My own menopausal journey has involved extraordinary moments of deep communion in the stillness enforced by weeks of sickening vertigo, and the most profound encounters with visionary dream spaces as I hid behind blinding headaches. I also began awakening early each dawn to the unsettling and often comical experience of dreaming in verse – and began to realize that as the flows of blood ceased, the flow of words increased. Each of these experiences has been helpfully put into the context of the great arc of the journey Kate describes, and I am grateful to her for her diligence and humour in revealing the vast territory of menopause, full of all us menopausal individuals, making our ways through the landscape of transformation, each of us making peace with ourselves and our own experiences.

Our life stories, our constitutions, our choices, and our cultural expectations all create a unique menopausal journey that calls each one of us to make peace with the lives we have lived so far, and to create the paths we shall walk in the future as the old women we are to become. Everyone's itinerary is different. And travelling without a map, it is so easy to get lost. Kate's brilliant book is an insightful and indispensable guide to the unfamiliar territory of menopause.

I give thanks and praise to Kate Codrington – the perfect travelling friend for us all as we navigate our own paths through menopause. This book is the ideal companion for a kick-ass menopause! Take courage from Kate's words, and let this journey of transformation be your own special time to find your way into a different flow – the flow of life's cycles through your unique emergence as you step into the fullness of your power postmenopause.

Uma Dinsmore-Tuli, PhD
Stroud, January 2022

Introduction

There has been a period revolution in my lifetime. When I had my first period it was a secret event, tainted with shame. At the time, the only menstrual product available was a giant pad held up with a peculiar contraption and safety pins. My daughter's generation has access to a wealth of information and can choose from a huge range of products: period pants, washable pads, cups, and disposable pads. Instead of something to be locked behind closed doors, we are owning the power of our menstruation, recognizing it as a multifaceted gift that adds creativity and depth to our lives. Menstrual shame is on the move. We are no longer 'cursed'.

Menopause is now on the cusp of a similar shift. As it slowly emerges from its place of shameful 'women's troubles', we now have menopause policies across all sectors, and it makes the main news on the television. While prominent women such as Kirsty Wark and Oprah Winfrey are talking publicly about their experience, most still hide symptoms or even take unpaid leave because menopause cannot be acknowledged if you want to be perceived as 'effective' at work. Many are forced to choose between demanding flexibility to create adjustments to their working life or having to leave the jobs they love because companies are not listening. Employers are slowly waking up to the expense of losing skilled women in their late forties, who were about to step into senior roles.

But like periods, menopause is more than a collection of physical events. It is also a psychological process that moves us into a new phase of our lives and can be an initiation into being our 'best self'. Menopause is, in fact, an inside job. You probably know about hot flushes, but the most powerful menopausal changes centre around your identity, who you are, and what kind of person you long to be. It can be a time of enormous growth and opportunity, which is followed by a Second Spring, as I'll be explaining in a little more detail soon.

'I LOVE MY POSTMENOPAUSAL LIFE!

FEWER CONCERNS, MORE OPENNESS.

LESS BULLSHIT.'

Liz

While the physical aspects, the flushes and aches and pains can be talked about fairly easily, the less visible psychological aspects can be unexpected and receive less care. As an initiation or rite of passage that moves us from one state of being to another, there is necessarily psychological pain. We can't get from our accommodating, mothering years to having a kick-ass Second Spring without fallout. This is normal. This *is* part of the process. God knows, we wish we could grow emotionally in an elegant style (keeping our good shoes unscuffed) but we all know that life doesn't work that way; we get knocked down, and we get up again. It's not pretty. It's much better than that. It's juicy. Luckily, despite the chaos there is an underlying organization that is moving us towards wholeness.

Like the Fairy Godmother of initiation, if you choose to engage consciously with the process, menopause can change you into the person you've always longed to be. You will enter your postmenopausal years not caring what others think, following what pleases you, full of vitality and able to use your 'no' wisely as you find your way towards greater fulfilment. The anthropologist Margaret Mead put it succinctly:

> *'There is no more creative force in the world than the menopausal woman with zest.'*[1]

I'm not saying it's easy, definitely not. You have likely grabbed this book because you feel like hell, are terrified that perimenopause is knocking on your door, or find yourself bang in the middle of it, and you're scared you're losing the plot or know someone who is. I am here to reassure you that if it's looking messy, then you're doing just fine. Menopause is a massive challenge, but it is also an initiation that can deliver you to a place of self-love that weeks of spa days will never get near.

About me

I have a confession: my name is Kate and I am addicted to personal growth. Or at least I was, until menopause came along and gifted me with a bespoke therapeutic experience to heal me good and proper.

I was an awkward teen, desperate to be cool, my appearance – partly shaved head and army fatigues – inadequately disguised my desperate need to be loved, to feel that I was OK. My big sister took me to one of those big 1980s' happy-clappy workshops with a room full of people weeping and despite my discomfort at the icky emotion (we weren't allowed to have feelings in our family), I began to wonder if maybe there was a way I could become more comfortable with myself – and so my addiction began. Receiving therapeutic massage was a revelation to me and started my journey to come into a better relationship with myself.

Along the way I have been gifted with some brilliant teachers. I learned biodynamic psychotherapy with Gerda Boyesen in the early 1990s. She was a trailblazer who pioneered the importance of stimulating the body's vagus nerve in healing and who, in the 1950s, highlighted the body's innate wisdom, long before this became mainstream. For many years I was a bodyworker, using massage, touch, and breathwork to help people heal their psychological wounds and feel better in themselves, including people with HIV and AIDS. After having my kids, now fabulous teenagers, I trained with Suzanne Yates at Wellmother, learning Shiatsu and movement for pregnancy, and this naturally led me to become awed at the power and magic of the womb. Training in womb massage followed as I deepened my understanding of women's reproductive health with leading yoga therapist Uma Dinsmore-Tuli and Alexandra Pope of Red School. My work life, when I'm not writing or chatting with interesting people for my podcast, is taken up with 1-2-1 mentoring, and groups and events that support people in menopause to develop a loving relationship with themselves and to trust that they are not broken and good times are ahead.

What this book will do

I'd love for this book to reassure you that menopause, far from wanting to destroy you, has your best interests at heart. Like a biological Miss Jean Brodie, she wants you to fulfil your full potential as a human so you can live the last third of your life as fully and creatively as possible. The book offers you a guide to the psychological phases of menopause, the low-down on how to manage the tricky physical challenges with lifestyle changes, and to understand what might be causing them. You'll get the truth about what HRT can do and a wealth of self-care practices created especially for menopause with which to soothe yourself and your symptoms. Understanding how to surf the wave of menopause will unlock the gifts of your Second Spring. Yes, there will be gifts!

Brain fog is a thing and what with everything else you've got going on, I get that there's not necessarily time to consume the whole book in one go. That's why it's divided into bite-sized sections so you can choose whether to go directly to whatever issue is hot for you right now, quickly understand what it's about, and choose a practice that will help you to manage your symptom better, or to read the chapters sequentially.

How the practices work

You'll find a range of practices for you to choose from, including a selection of journaling prompts, small lifestyle changes, yoga nidra (a form of guided meditation), tweaks to your diet, and all kinds of other things that you are welcome to take or leave as you choose. As the process of menopause brings you into your own authority, you get to choose what works and what doesn't, and the practices serve to shine light on the resources you already have.

As well as being right here at your fingertips, as a *Second Spring* bonus, you can also download audio versions of some of the features, such as the yoga nidras and meditations, at katecodrington.co.uk/second-spring-downloads/. There are numerous suggestions for exploration and small changes in these pages and on my website, so I invite you to take things at your own pace and in your own way. This is not an improvement programme and you cannot get this wrong!

Before taking on any of the practices, check in with your body: does thinking about that practice make you feel more relaxed and better in yourself, or more tense and pressured? It's so easy to fall for what we think we ought to do, and then when we can no longer push ourselves to do the miserable thing, feel disappointed that we have 'failed'. Only do what feels good for as long as it feels good.

Please do your own research into the suggestions I offer and be aware that some seemingly innocent herbal remedies can react badly with medications. You are responsible for your wellbeing. Always speak to your doctor in case of doubt. I hope the tools and inspiration will help you discover greater kindness for yourself and to realize, finally, that you don't need fixing at all. You are fully empowered to take what you need and ditch the rest.

Sometimes life is so intense that even one small practice is too much, so when you're completely frazzled, a reminder that you're doing OK is handy. That's why each topic is closed with a little phrase to capture the essence of the care you can give yourself. Often irreverent and light-hearted, these little mantras will wave a flag and help raise a smile when things get tough. If you find one that grabs you, you are welcome to jot it down on a Post-it Note or your screen saver to help guide you through your day.

Quotes

All through the book you'll find quotes from ordinary people describing their experiences. My intention is to show you that you are not alone, that all across the world we are journeying through the choppy seas together, and that you will be OK. I've been gifted with stories of release and redemption from my interviewees in perimenopause and menopause, telling it like it is, and from those in Second Spring who have the advantage of perspective as they look back at their menopause experience. Like big sisters, they show us the way forward. I also plagued my friends and community with endless questions about their menopause experiences, which they were kind enough to answer and allow to be published and shared with you here. Where I've quoted someone who preferred to be anonymous, I've changed their name and put it in inverted commas.

There is nothing as inspiring to me as the power of (extra)ordinary people's stories of healing and pulling through after life has side-swiped them. Time after time, I am moved to tears as people see that they are much more than they thought, that there are riches and joy to be had despite, or even because of, the wounding they received. It's an absolute privilege to be trusted with these unfolding narratives, and this book has been written by the clients and retreat participants who have been generous enough to share their stories. I am indebted to you all.

The Seasons

The book is all about the Seasons of your life and how, by listening kindly to your body's needs, you can understand for yourself what remedies will support your healing. Like the rhythms of the year, our inner Life Seasons invite us to be more active and venture out into the world in Spring and Summer, followed by quieter and more sensitive time in Autumn and Winter. This is true of our daily rhythm and the menstrual cycle, and also in our lives, with Inner Spring being the teens and twenties years from the time of our first period, Summer in our thirties, Autumn bringing perimenopause, Winter deep menopause, and then – *tada!* – Second Spring! A whole new cycle of expansion. In traditional Chinese medicine, Second Spring is the time after menopause that is characterized by a renewed and expansive vitality. Postmenopausal life is a rebirth, bringing a Second Spring full of new possibilities.

'I NO LONGER CARE WHAT ANYONE THINKS, I AM FINALLY FREE!'

'Clare'

The trouble comes – trouble meaning menopause symptoms – when we ignore the call to 'stay home' and continue to pretend that it's Summer when the leaves have fallen in Autumn and Winter.

In tandem with these Seasons, you will also find a psychological map for the menopause process: Separation, Surrender, and Emergence[2]. The first part of the process, perimenopause or Separation, invites us to slow down and release what no longer serves us. This usually hurts. A lot. Wounds and trauma we have shoved under the carpet for years emerge for healing. The physical symptoms of menopause are asking us to slow down, inviting us to listen to our bodies and respond kindly. In our culture, we tend to respond to this by sticking our fingers in our ears and humming. But menopause keeps knocking on our door until we listen, trying to help us to release cumbersome identities and roles, and this requires space and slowing down. Ultimately, menopause encourages us to release old patterns and step forwards naked as we birth ourselves into the unknown, to find a new and more authentic way of being.

Surrender, the second phase, is all about acceptance and building a relationship with yourself. This is the point at which you can allow yourself to say no to things, to coast a bit, rest more, and really engage with the kind of restful things that nourish you. If you think of the pleasures of annual winter – a roaring fire, soft cosy socks and warming soup – you'll get the feeling of Surrender.

Emergence, the third phase, is when you start to entertain the possibility of venturing into the world again as ideas and possibilities arrive for your attention. Your challenge at this time is to receive and allow yourself to fill without giving your energy away by rushing out and muscling through. Rest and withdrawal are so counter-cultural that it's hard to allow ourselves to put off our to-do lists and obligations for so long, but it is *so* worth it!

'I FEEL WISE, POWERFUL,

CONFIDENT, INTOLERANT OF CRAP

AND CERTAINLY NOT INVISIBLE.'

Catherine

I appreciate that all of this might be new information to you, and that you might feel sceptical at the idea of postmenopausal life being vibrant and creative. Luckily for you I have included a Menstruality Medicine Circle process, which will give you an embodied experience of how the Seasons and phases work to renew you into a new, lighter way of being. It is a safe way to access your own unique path to your understanding and self-care for physical, mental, and spiritual wellbeing. You can find out more about them in chapter 16.

A collaboration

This book would not exist without the Seasonal map of menstruation and the phases of menopause that have their origins in the pioneering work of Red School, founded by Alexandra Pope and Sjanie Hugo Wurlitzer. Alexandra, also known as the 'Red Pope', is my favourite kind of person, responsible for a ton of original concepts and over forty years of activism that have changed the experience of menstruation and menopause in the West. Suffering from extreme menstrual pain in her thirties, she decided to forgo painkillers and the medical treatment offered, and decided instead to follow her instinct to go inwards, listening to what her body was trying to tell her. While she was ridiculed by the press for many years for proclaiming the power and wisdom of the menstrual cycle, the world has finally caught up with her in the last few years. Together with Sjanie, she co-founded Red School to educate and support feminine leadership, and co-wrote *Wild Power*, which I strongly recommend you read.

It was from these awesome women that I learned the art of the Menstruality Medicine Circle, adapted into the Circle process in these pages. After nearly thirty years of professional experience, I have never come across any process as gentle and profound as the Circles; they are pure magic. I owe Sjanie and Alexandra a deep debt of gratitude for their profound teachings and care, and for allowing me to include the Circle process in this book.

The third person who has been pivotal is my dear friend Leora Leboff, who is a menstrual and menopause mentor, and womb massage practitioner. We have worked, laughed, and learned together in close partnership since 2014, offering online and in-person retreats as Woman Kind. Through our own lived experience of the menopause process and that of our clients, we have simplified the phases to make them more accessible and adapted the Circles to match. Leora's wisdom, deep thinking, and her patience with me is woven into every page.

Put these three nourishing, savoury women into the pot, and stir in my work in complementary therapy with my wonderful clients, and you get *Second Spring*. I am hugely grateful for all that these extraordinary people have gifted me.

Because this body of information has grown from my work with largely cisgendered women, the book reflects that. Not everyone who has menopause is a woman; trans men, non-binary, genderfluid and intersex folk also experience menopause and there is a desperate need for guides to menopause transition accessible for all people. As far as I can tell there is no research done on this area at all and what support does exist, is limited to peer support groups. I'm aware that this is a charged topic on all sides and my heartfelt wish is that all those going through menopause will access space and support to make the transition in their own way. Attitudes are changing fast, and I can only share things as they are in the here and now. I am greatly indebted to the trans and non-binary folk who trusted me enough to share their stories about menopause, and I am greatly honoured to include them here. My intention is to open the conversation about the transformational possibilities of menopause to include more voices. If you have a story you think should be heard, you can contact me through my website.

Though our experiences are unique, the three psychological phases of change – Separation, Surrender, and Emergence – are universal. These phases map the process of bereavement, illness or spiritual awakening, a shift in consciousness, and they're familiar to every human. I hope that however you identify, however you love, and whatever your culture, understanding more about these phases will be helpful. The most powerful action you could take in perimenopause (or bereavement, illness or breakdown) might be just to name Separation, and in that recognition, remember that you are not falling apart even though it feels like you are; you are in a place of growth and need a little more space to do that. Helena Bonham Carter reminds us of the rewards that await:

> *'Why can't we be sexually and romantically attractive when our eggs are expired? Actually, it's much more fun because we're so freed of the terror, there is no consequence, it's all just for fun.'*[3]

I use the word 'woman' a lot because the experiences I have witnessed and describe here have mostly happened to people who identify as women. It would be over-performative to use language that does not describe the people I have mostly worked with. If you find this disrespectful, I can only apologize.

'WE'RE THE ONES WE'VE BEEN
WAITING FOR.'

June Jordan, 'Poem for South African Women'[4]

You don't need fixing,
you really don't.

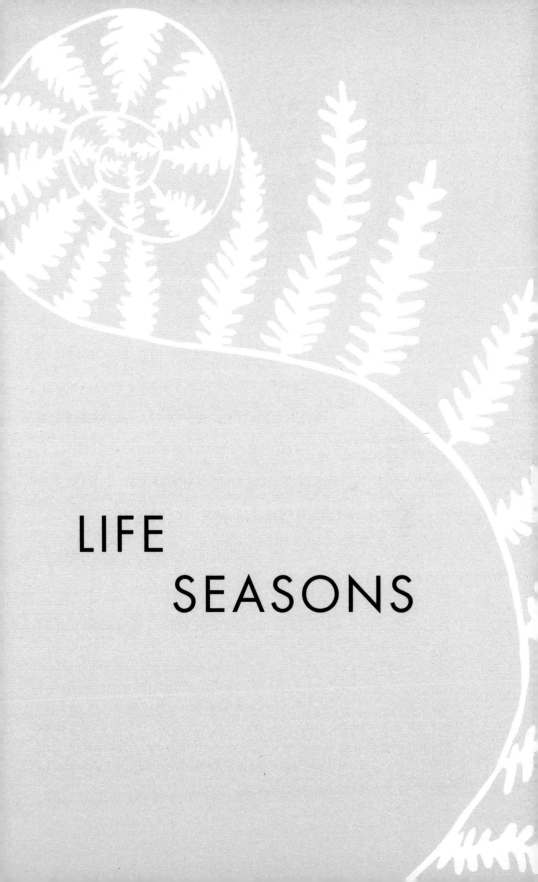

LIFE
SEASONS

1 The Life Seasons

'SEEING THE SEASONS WITHIN
SWITCHED ON A LIGHT BULB IN
MY HEAD. USING THE LANDSCAPE
OF SEASONS TOOK ME OUT OF
THE NEGATIVITY OF SOCIETY'S
SHRIVELLED PERCEPTION OF
MENOPAUSE AND GAVE ME THE
POWER TO HAVE CONFIDENCE
AND TRUST IN MYSELF. I COULD
FLOURISH IN MY SECOND SPRING.'

Kate T.

The idea that there are different Seasons in life offers an incredibly helpful way to understand ourselves at different ages, and the various experiences that we are likely to encounter. Each Life Season has a 'developmental task', a psychological step to be taken to move towards wholeness.[1] Just like the annual seasons, this is a cyclical process, and there are no hard and fast rules: in the same way that the year's seasons may vary, with an unexpectedly cold spring or a wonderfully sunny autumn, so can individual experiences of these Inner Life Seasons vary from person to person. This is why I'd like to start by exploring their significance and the phases of menopause associated with them, so you can get a feel for the natural rhythm this creates and what it might mean in your own life.

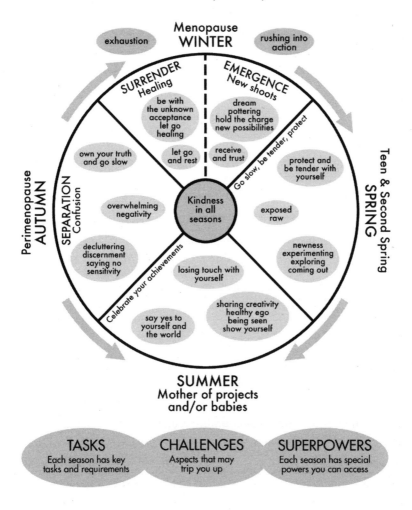

LIFE SEASONS
Each season represents a stage of a woman's life from menarche to postmenopause

The circle of the Seasons of Life

(created in collaboration with Leora Leboff)

Life Spring

Menarche is your first period. It's the start of Life Spring, and it brings boundless energy, exploration, and the vulnerability of youth. We are feeling our way into the world and exploring who we might become; we're tender, just like emerging buds. Being held back or wounded in our Spring, as many of us are, has a lifelong effect on the way we approach each Season that follows. The developmental tasks of Life Spring are to explore and to play while protected by our family and culture.

Life Summer

The Summer Season of life is where we blossom our creativity into the world, maybe by having children, in work, or through creative or community projects. A time of healthy ego, we take our essence and shape it into real constructs in the outside world. Just as in annual summer, we want to be out there partying with our people, so it is in this Life Summer; it might be both thrilling and overwhelming to be pulled 'out there' into the world. The developmental tasks are to express your spirit in the world and say a resounding YES to yourself and to life.

Life Autumn and Separation

The crossover from Summer to Autumn represents the shift to perimenopause and the beginning of greater sensitivity; this shades into Separation, the first phase of menopause. In the same way as the nights become noticeably longer in October, we are pulled away from the outside world to look inwards and become more reflective. The leaves have fallen to reveal the shape of the trees, and we start to see things much more clearly. We become more discerning and are unafraid to tell people about what we see, often with the volume turned up to eleven. Separation can be a long, hard haul, especially when we resist it; we may feel like we're losing the plot.

It is, essentially, the hurty bit. Though it can be a deeply uncomfortable time, it is corrective; this inward-looking energy counterbalances the decades of outward business. We are required to take our foot off the gas and just slow down. Separation shows us our vulnerabilities and sensitivity, in health and our lives, asking us to listen and tend to ourselves gently. One woman mentioned that she developed a 'heavy, catastrophic' way of thinking completely out of nowhere, not triggered by anything in particular; another described a 'sense of gloom' – and both required great tenderness and care. Sudden impatience and irritability are almost universal in Separation, because it is a sensitive time when we see what is wrong. You are not going mad: the Autumn and Separation bring the shadows into the light, and the parts of ourselves that are not integrated are showing up. You'll still be having periods in Separation, and they might be changing from your normal pattern. The developmental tasks are to discern your truth within yourself and your world, and to stay kind and present.

Life Winter, Surrender, and Emergence

Life Winter is the time of deep menopause, and has two phases that shade into each other. The first phase is Surrender, the point at which you start to accept the changes in yourself, begin to engage with healing and refill your tanks. It feels a little easier, not because the challenges have gone away, but because you've come to accept them more and let go of the urgency to fix everything. Like annual winter, it calls us to be quiet, stay close to home, to rest, and receive. It's a time when we have easy access to our spirituality and intuition. Spend enough time resting and healing in Surrender and you'll find yourself in Emergence, the second Wintery phase, when ideas about possibilities for new ways of being and projects will start to form. Your challenge here is to receive the ideas and the new energy for yourself without giving it away. At some point in your Life Winter your periods will stop for good. The developmental tasks of Winter are to let go and rest in Surrender, and to receive and trust in Emergence.

Second Spring and the new cycle

Second Spring equates to postmenopause and is a potent time, the beginning of a whole new cycle. You'll know you're there because you have an internal sense of having arrived somewhere; you feel the absence of change. It continues the Emergence phase you started in your Life Winter, a gradual process of coming back out into the world as your energy builds. It's a bit like the annual spring in that you can sense in the air that new life is coming even before you see it. Gradually, the new ideas and possibilities start to take shape containing all the best qualities of your first Life Spring, including vulnerability and experimentation, but this time round with the wisdom gained from difficult life lessons learned and a big dose of *don't give a shit*. The developmental tasks of Second Spring are to explore and to be tender with yourself.

'I FINALLY GET TO BE THE
TEENAGER I LONGED TO BE ALL
THOSE YEARS AGO.'

Fern

Second Summer

After our tender arrival in Second Spring, in Second Summer we find our feet, put on our boots, and get walking Nancy Sinatra style. This time in our sixties and early seventies packs a powerhouse of wisdom and resolve, where once again – whether it's conquering new loves for mountain climbing or grandchildren – we are manifesting our unique contributions to the world 'out there'. Sceptical that this is all too much woo? Data from half a million Americans and Europeans showed that happiness is 'U'-shaped: as we head into our fifties, levels of contentment rise so that by the time we're in our sixties, it's likely that we'll never have been happier.[2]

Second Autumn

This 'U'-curve continues into the following Seasons, where one study found that 82 was the age of maximum happiness.[3] This Season sees another round of letting go as we face our mortality, releasing our grip on material things, and retreat inwards, reflecting on what has been important in our lives and what might need closure.

Second Winter

The final Season of our lives, in this Winter we harvest the wisdom gathered in all the other smaller Winters of our lives – menstruation, annual winter, menopause – and prepare to say goodbye to our time on earth.

*

So how does this Seasonal structure work in real life, with real people and all the stuff that life throws at us? We all have different life experiences, after all. The Seasons and phases show the 'natural order' of an uninterrupted life, which no one ever has! But we feel these internal movements towards exploring in spring, manifesting in summer, etc. as internal pressure, perhaps most especially when they are frustrated. Our wounding or setback in one Season will impact how fully we can inhabit the others. Each Season has its own developmental tasks and where we skip one, it tends to show up later to be completed. Think of the goody-goody head girl who goes bat-shit-crazy for partying in her thirties, for example. Or the blossoming satisfaction in pursuing career goals, only to find you forgot to have a child.

As a late developer, I had a very long Life Spring trying to wriggle out from my family's expectations and figure out who the hell I really was (featuring a neon-orange, cornrowed Mohican at one time, sucking up ALL the cultural appropriation on one head!), and then squished my Life Summer into a couple of years when I squeezed out a couple of kids, dumping all the chaos and activity of Life Summer into my Life Autumn. The Summery need to express my spirit in the world through my work and children, when combined and layered over the Autumnal desire to slow down and retreat, created conflicting needs and it was quite a challenge. Babies + perimenopause – support = messy. It's important to know that the perfectly unfolding Seasonal life *does not exist*, but understanding the qualities and developmental tasks associated with each Season is super helpful to unpick the conflicts you're experiencing, and how best to take care of yourself.

The Seasons are phases are felt within you and are not tightly bound up with the physicality of menopause, but broadly you could say that you will still have periods in Separation, but by the time you come to Emergence, you will have stopped.

For those using artificial hormones, whether for birth control, to manage their menopause symptoms or to align their gender, the Seasons and phases may be less pronounced and you may not feel so much urgency within the cycle. Nevertheless, being human, you are governed by these cycles and understanding the structure will help you unlock more healing and creativity.

The Seasons of your menstrual cycle itself – the Summer of ovulation, Autumn of the premenstruum, Winter of menstruation and Spring of post-menstruation – can be used as a rehearsal for the themes and challenges of menopause. If the Autumn of perimenopause seems familiar to you, it's probably because you've lived it for a week or so every month of your adult life. The same themes and triggers that pop up in your premenstrual phase and during your period will be coming up even louder and stronger and for longer in your Life Autumn and Winter. The good news is, if you still have a cycle, you get to hone your awareness and self-care skills every month. Menstrual Autumn and Winter can show you the way to your resources in perimenopause. Even if you don't have a menstrual cycle now, you might like to take time to look back and reflect on how it was for you in the past.

PRACTICE

Here are some journaling prompts to use to access your self-help skills:

- In my premenstrual phase, what got to me was ...
- To soothe myself in my premenstrual phase I would use ...
- When I have/had my period I would love to ...

Relax into the flow of life.

2 The basics

Menopause lasts a moment, but perimenopause lasts a long, long time. Let me explain. Perimenopause means that you have menopausal symptoms; it's the change in your hormones as you gradually move towards your last period. Many clients have told me that they 'knew' something was up, even when their doctor said it couldn't be perimenopause. Generally, perimenopause might start in your late thirties or early forties, and its arrival can be obvious for some, or you might not be aware of it at all. Perimenopause is a sensitive time, like puberty, and underlying health issues often show up. Used less often, the term 'climacteric' means the broad time of perimenopause and postmenopause.

Menopause happens when it's been a year since your last period, and after that you're postmenopausal, so technically menopause is only a moment long. It usually occurs between the ages of 45 and 55 years, unless you have a surgical menopause where your womb and ovaries are removed, or a chemical menopause, following cancer treatment, for example. Early menopause, before 45, affects approximately 5 per cent of the population. The time drawing towards your last period is called perimenopause and afterwards you are postmenopausal. Sounds so straightforward, doesn't it?

The hottest question I'm asked is 'Am I in perimenopause?' and these basic descriptions don't really answer that; in fact there is an infinitely wide range of experiences, most of which are 'normal'. Almost all symptoms are exacerbated by stress, fear of ageing, and toxicity in food or your environment. Ever seen those towels that are hung up to celebrate Towel Day as a tribute to Douglas Adams's novel *The Hitchhiker's Guide to the Galaxy*? They say 'DON'T PANIC' in large friendly letters. For a similar fix, try out the practice below.

PRACTICE

- Take a pause just for a moment, wherever you are. Become aware of the places your body touches your support, your seat or the floor.
- Try pushing your feet into the ground or wiggling your bum to sensitize yourself to the contact you are making with your surroundings.
- Notice your breath as it moves through you. The feel of your clothes and the air on your skin. Any smells or taste in your mouth.
- Become aware of the sounds around you. What colours and shapes do you see? Be here now.
- Ask yourself: What do I *really* need right now?

There is only this moment.

3 It's your hormones

It's useful to understand a bit about how hormones work, because this knowledge can empower you to become the authority on yourself and reduce feelings of helplessness. Understanding how the fluctuations in the body's endocrine system affect you will help you find treatment and practise self-care, as well as reassuring you that you're not going mad. Knowledge is indeed power. I would be cautious, though, not to get lost in overthinking: frantic Googling about brain fog is not going to help you think more clearly, and will probably raise your anxiety. Splitting body and mind into two separate categories is like reducing an extraordinarily profound system into a Ford Capri – when we do this we can miss out on the real juice of wellbeing. Rather than being made up of mechanical bits and bobs, you are comprised of interconnected systems in a dynamic state of flux. As Liz Koch explains in *Stalking Wild Psoas*:

> *Now is the time to dissolve the old story and inhabit the new paradigm of body as a living process.*[1]

Your first step in finding help should always be 'What kindness can I show myself now?' before anything else happens. However, by understanding the hormone picture at menopause, you can access further self-help for your challenges.

For the years of your menstruating life, your hormones oestrogen and progesterone perform a beautiful dance together to create your menstrual cycle. These hormones dance to the symphony of the wondrously complex and subtle endocrine system, which governs pretty much every function in your body. You tweak one bit of the system and all your body's systems are affected.

Introducing your friendly hormones

Oestrogen is the stuff that makes us curvy and caring. It builds up the lining of the womb to make a comfy home for an egg to implant into, protects against bone loss, keeps your blood vessels healthy, affects your serotonin levels and your mood, and gives you plump skin and a juicy vagina.

Progesterone maintains the womb lining, so it's high throughout pregnancy to support a good supply of blood to the womb. It also plays a part in bone health, soothes you and helps you to sleep, manages your food cravings, appetite and energy, and it has an anti-inflammatory effect.

Follicle-stimulating hormone and luteinizing hormone work together in the menstrual cycle. Follicle-stimulating hormone triggers the ovarian follicles to ripen your eggs, while luteinizing hormone triggers the eggs to pop out at ovulation and then nudges the corpus luteum in the ovary to produce progesterone in the second half of your cycle.

Testosterone is also a player in menopause; it supports your libido, maintains energy levels, and can be converted into oestrogen. Fun fact: in our menstruating years we have three times as much testosterone as oestrogen, and this declines as we age.

The hormones involved in the fight-or-flight response are adrenaline, which takes care of the initial reaction to the trigger, and cortisol, which kicks in a few minutes later. Cortisol plays a role in our menopausal dance, because if you have chronic stress – like when you're worrying about work, the kids, the environment, and whether you're good enough for twenty years straight – your body continuously produces cortisol, which contributes to all kinds of problems. Both are made in the adrenal glands, which also produce our precious supplies of oestrogen in Second Spring; if you've knackered your adrenal glands already, you'll be in for a hard time during perimenopause, with physical and emotional symptoms.

*

Here's a 'typical' pattern of hormone change through Separation and all the way to Second Spring. When I say 'typical' it's like a driver's seat in the car: it fits almost nobody; we will all have our own unique hormonal issues that we inherit or acquire through our lives.

As you move through your forties towards perimenopause, your hormonal balance will change as your ovaries slow their production of both oestrogen and progesterone; it's not necessarily a tidy, polite decline, though. While progesterone generally declines at an even rate, there are often spikes of oestrogen highs and lows, where the dance can become wilder, often in the space of a day. This is where oestrogen dominance can occur, meaning that it is relatively high compared to the level of progesterone. This is very common and can happen either because chronic stress has lowered your progesterone or there are too many xenoestrogens – compounds that mimic the effects of oestrogen or promote its production – around you in plastics or food. (See chapter 31 for more on these.) Because oestrogen is also produced in fat cells, being overweight can also contribute to oestrogen dominance. There is a relationship between oestrogen dominance and hypothyroidism, which might show up as tiredness, weight gain or depression, symptoms that are interchangeable with menopause issues.[2]

It's interesting to note that for people who experience PMT, it's not so much that their hormones are out of balance but that they are highly hormone-sensitive. A sensitivity to progesterone seems to reduce serotonin, the neurotransmitter that helps to regulate mood. Unfortunately, there is some correlation between those who have experienced PMDD (premenstrual dysphoric disorder) and postnatal depression and difficulty at menopause. This is useful to recognize so that if you are one of them, you can be super kind to yourself and plan extra measures and support to manage your sensitivity.

Once the ovaries stop releasing eggs altogether, they produce much less oestrogen and no progesterone. Now that the levels of these two hormones are low, the lining of the uterus no longer builds up and menstruation stops, until you finally forget all about that bleeding business and realize you've arrived in a different country: Second Spring. If you have a bleed of any kind once you are postmenopausal, more than a year after your last period, it's good to check with your doctor as it can be an indication of endometrial cancer.

In your Second Spring, you'll have the same follicle-stimulating hormone and luteinizing hormone levels as before puberty. It is generally said that this is the body's attempt to kick-start ovulation, but this seems to be faulty thinking; surely our bodies are more efficient than that? In her seminal book *The Wisdom of Menopause*, women's health maven Dr Christiane Northrup suggests that these high levels serve as extra neuro-transmitters on the right side of the brain, increasing creativity, intuition, and visionary experiences.[3] It's the Second Spring vibe: the mentality of curiosity and exploration we had as a girl returns, but thankfully this time with added 'fuckitall' – the secret ingredient for a spicy third age.

Postmenopause, it's our ovaries, adrenals, and most of all our body fat that handles our oestrogen production in the form of estrone. This is why being a stressed-out Second Springer with a low-BMI can be problematic, because having low body fat and tired adrenals will floor your oestrogen levels completely and can put your long-term health at risk, affecting your bone health in particular as well as leading to low moods. There is a well-known saying attributed to Catherine Deneuve about midlife body fat: 'You have to choose between your face and your ass.' But for health, perhaps it could be said you have to choose between your arse and your bones, as having a low BMI postmenopause increases the risk of osteoporosis.[4]

It's worth making a big out-shout here to your liver, which filters the blood from the digestive tract – thereby not only handling vats of prosecco but also playing a big role in hormone regulation. It works as a processor that regulates and eliminates excess hormones, especially oestrogen; creates specific proteins that act as hormone carriers; and plays a role in manufacturing testosterone and oestrogen, as well as producing bile to break down and eliminate other toxins. Whether it's dealing with the hormones your body has produced or HRT, the liver hoovers up and deals with the excess – so if it's overworked by its other tasks, the hormone regulation part of its job will be impaired.

The following info can give you some insight into where your hormones could do with a tweak and what lifestyle measures might be useful to think about.

Self-help for hormones at a glance

If you are concerned about your health, please consult your doctor or physician for professional medical advice. The recommendations in this table are only guidelines and not intended as a diagnostic tool.

Hormonal imbalance	Possible signs include:	If this looks like a pattern for you, try:
High cortisol	• Feeling wired and tired • Sleep issues • Feeling tense • Anxiety and feeling nervy • Quickly running to anger • A cuddly muffin top • Sugar cravings • Feeling or being judged as thin-skinned • Getting shaky between meals	• Resting more • Doing a stress audit on your life to examine what's winding you up most and what you can change • A mindful practice such as yoga nidra, meditation or a breath practice • Find things that soothe you • Slowing everything down • Drinking less coffee, Coke and tea • Adding maca powder into your diet (see page 45)
Low cortisol (aka prolonged stress)	• Burnout • A 2pm energy crash • Feeling weepy and feeble • Getting easily overwhelmed • Hyper-sensitivity emotionally • Sleep issues • Getting sweaty more easily • Experiencing unexpected joint pain, unrelated to anything else • Dizziness	• Getting more rest • Finding enjoyable movement • Finding a routine that enhances the circadian rhythm • Getting out into the sunshine, especially in the mornings • Letting go of goals, 'shoulds' and 'oughts' • Adopting a breath practice • Drinking less coffee, tea, and Coke • Adding maca powder into your diet (see page 45)

Hormonal imbalance	Possible signs include:	If this looks like a pattern for you, try:
Low progesterone	• Anxiety • Food cravings, especially carbs and sugar • Endometriosis • Less frequent and heavier periods • Headaches • Migraine • Water retention • Cysts • Restless legs, especially at night	• Leaning more into your friendships and support networks • More orgasms! • Drinking less booze and coffee • Eat dark chocolate • Using castor oil packs (see page 47) • Also have a look at the self-care for oestrogen dominance, below
Excess oestrogen, aka oestrogen dominance	• Low energy • Low libido • Headaches • Anxiety • High tension generally • Sore boobs • Rapid weight gain despite eating well • Fibroids • Worsening PMS	• Heaping on the self-kindness • Letting go of your guilt • Increasing the nutrients in your diet • Doing a stress audit on your life to examine what's winding you up most and what you can change • Increasing vitamin P, aka pleasure! • Reducing xenoestrogens (see chapter 31) • Reducing caffeine and booze • Add a few prunes and some turmeric to your diet • Show your liver some love with extra whole grains and vegetables • Try a castor oil pack on your liver (see page 47) • Try supplementing with DIM supplements (see page 45)
Low oestrogen	• Brain fog • Flushing • Night sweats • Dry skin and vagina • Bladder issues • Depression • Lighter periods • Achy joints or injuries	• Avoiding caffeine and gluten • Adding flaxseed to your diet • More orgasms (hooray!) • Gentle exercise • Eating fresh pomegranate • Taking vitamin E • Using sea buckthorn supplements • Upping magnesium from almonds, cashews and black beans • Using maca power (see page 45) in your smoothies or sweet treats

Hormonal imbalance	Possible signs include:	If this looks like a pattern for you, try:
Excess androgens	• Excess body and facial hair • Greasy hair and skin • Skin tags • Thinning hair on head • Longer cycles • Ovarian cysts • Polycystic ovarian syndrome (PCOS)	• Vibrant, aerobic exercise • Reduce or cut out refined carbs and sugar • Eat more fibrous foods such as legumes and whole grains • Snack on sesame or tahini and pumpkin seeds • Consume less dairy and more protein • Sprinkle food with cinnamon • Go to a regular yoga class
Low thyroid	• Dry skin and brittle nails • Fluid retention (puffy ankles or knees) • Feeling cold all the time • Noticing slow speech and a slow brain to match • Fatigue and exhaustion • Heavy periods • Low libido • Depression	• Being super tender towards yourself • Doing a stress audit on your life to examine what's winding you up most and what you can change • Expressing your feelings safely • Finding a kind of exercise that makes you happy • Eating more seaweed, dates, macadamia nuts, walnuts, and dairy • Taking up meditation, yoga nidra or breathwork • Cognitive behavioural therapy (CBT)
Low testosterone	• Low libido • Brain fog • Depression • Fatigue • Weight gain	• Lifting weights • Eating more protein • Eating more healthy fats like olive oil avocados and nuts • Adding more healthy carbs to your diet • Doing a stress audit on your life to examine what's winding you up most and what you can change • Getting out in the sunshine • Resting more • Reducing xenoestrogens

Before you make any changes at all, ask yourself, 'How can I be kinder to myself right now?' and see what comes up, and keep on asking it through your day. You are a beautifully complex magical miracle just in and of yourself, and reducing guilt, judgement, and self-hatred will lessen the pressure of the stress you put yourself under, which will improve your symptoms. This is always the best way to start.

Be aware that with the choppy seas of menopause, many factors might be at play, so when you are considering making changes in your diet or lifestyle, it's most helpful to make one small change at a time for a few weeks and monitor your symptoms. It's too easy to make changes in a punitive way, which just re-enforces self-hatred and misery, so please make your changes kindly, take pleasure and in your new habits, and give them to yourself as you would to a beloved friend. Keeping a journal or diary is really helpful to keep track of what's going on – especially with brain fog, when you've no clue what you started when or what the hell happened this morning. Of course, in real life we have an ever-changing selection of symptoms that are like a hormonal pick-and-mix from this table. If this is the case for you, try to identify what's bothering you most and track that.

You can also see if the following two food supplements are helpful:

Maca is a relative of broccoli that grows high up in the Andes in Peru. The ground root has a pleasing malty flavour to it and though there's limited research, it appears that its high nutritional value can be of benefit and it's generally used to balance the hormones as well as to increase libido.

DIM contains a component of cruciferous veggies called diindolylmethane, which has an effect like eating a truckload of broccoli, only without the wind. There's a link in the Resources on page 396 if you want to find out more.

Keep your liver happy too

Many of us report, with sadness, that even a small glass of wine sends us over the edge. Perhaps this is the body's way of sharing its needs, because your liver has to work hard to neutralize the effects of alcohol. Cut back on the booze and your liver will thank you.

No surprise that caffeine and processed food will also put strain on your liver, but don't forget that environmental toxins also have to be processed within the body (see chapter 31). If you're already eating well enough, what can you add in to support it? Try these:

- Stay hydrated with water.
- Broccoli helps the liver to produce enzymes that clear the toxins.
- Beetroot enhances liver function.
- Lentils help with their lovely fibre.
- Lemons are great for supporting digestion.
- Apples – one a day really might keep the doctor away.
- Onions and garlic contain the compound allicin, which helps the liver and nourishes the blood.

What kindness can I show myself right now?

Castor Oil Pack

Castor oil packs are a low-cost, simple way of promoting good circulation and a gentle detox, usually used on either the liver or the lower abdomen. You might be familiar with castor oil as something to get your bowels moving; rest assured this is altogether gentler. To use the warmed oil over the womb or liver is an ancient, traditional remedy and while there's not been much research into the benefits, it has proved anecdotally helpful for perimenopause and menopause. It's particularly useful for common issues such as:

- fibroids
- ovarian cysts
- endometriosis
- abdominal pain

The combination of the oil and the warmth supports the circulation and can also dramatically reduce internal and external scarring.[5] Using it on the area above your liver will support hormone balance and, of course, lying down all cosy and warm is just a wonderful moment to give yourself.

CAUTIONS

It's important to start slowly with castor oil packs, and if you have unwanted symptoms afterwards to reduce the time or stop using them altogether. Make sure to stay hydrated and drink an extra glass or water or two when you do use them.

Do not use castor oil packs if you have:

- high blood pressure
- your period
- an acute or suspected digestive condition
- suspected but as yet undiagnosed tumours

or

- if pregnant

unless under the supervision of an appropriately trained professional.

WHEN AND HOW OFTEN

- For an acute situation, use them three times a week.
- Start with ten minutes and build up time if your body responds well.
- If you want to conceive, then only in the first half of your cycle, before you ovulate.
- It's wise to be careful if you use them while you're bleeding; although some people like them, heat can make heavy bleeding worse.

WHAT YOU'LL NEED

- a bottle of castor oil, preferably organic
- a flannel, old bit of towel or a muslin baby square
- a hot water bottle or heat pad – but *not too hot or you'll scald yourself*
- a second muslin square or old small towel to cover the pack while you're using it
- old clothes to wear and an old towel to lie on, because castor oil will stain
- a glass jar or lidded container to store the oil in between sessions
- baking soda to help wash off the oil afterwards

WHAT TO DO

- Fold your flannel so it's the right size for the area you're treating.
- Put it into your glass container (you'll probably have to fold it some more) and pour in the oil so it saturates the cloth. Poking it about a bit helps. The oil gets much runnier when it's warmed so don't use too much.
- Armed with the rest of the equipment from the list above, find somewhere comfy and lie down on your old towel.
- Take your oil-saturated cloth and place it over your liver (right side of bottom ribs and waist) or lower abdomen if it's for your womb, and cover it with the second, clean muslin or small towel.
- Pop your hot water bottle or heat pad on top.
- Relax and read your book, meditate, snooze or whatever pleases you.
- Afterwards, replace the oily cloth in the glass container.
- Wipe off any excess oil. A little baking soda in warm water will do the trick.
- You can re-use the pack up to five times.

If you're using castor oil packs for a particular issue, do it three times a week for a month and then review to see if it has helped. It's also great to use in combination with the Self-Care Abdominal Massage (see pages 74–76 for instructions).

4 A horrible history of menopause

I hope that you're sitting comfortably and have your smelling salts to hand: the history of how menopause has been treated is not pretty. Nearly everything documented about menopause has been written by men[1], most of it misogynistic, but if you think things are bad now, then this horrible history might give you some rather alarming perspective.

Around the time of the Bronze Age, at the dawn of the patriarchal system, menopause started to be pathologized as a dysfunction. In ancient Greece, Aristotle, who, safe to say, was probably not a feminist, came up with the diagnosis of the 'wandering womb', which was the origin of the many and varied invasive procedures that followed. It wasn't until 1821 that French physician Charles Pierre Louis de Gardanne coined the term 'la ménépausie'. What his wife called it before then has not been recorded.

In 1710, it was considered a disease but by the nineteenth century this had escalated to an all-out crisis. Hysterectomies, ovary removal, and even clitorectomies were widespread as a cure for all sorts of ailments ascribed to la ménépausie. According to Louise Foxcroft in her book Hot Flushes, Cold Science,[2] hysteria, alcoholism, nymphomania (aka those who had the indecency to enjoy their sexual lives), being 'stridently manly', and even spontaneous combustion have all considered menopausal symptoms at one time or another. With surgery in its infancy and anaesthesia not yet invented, there was a monstrously high mortality rate. Other remedies included an aperitif of carbonated soda, a belladonna plaster to the pit of the stomach, vaginal injections containing acetate of lead, or being locked up in an asylum with a diagnosis of 'climactic insanity'. No wonder we were hysteric alcoholics. For the less adventurous physicians, opium, morphine, and chloric ether were popular choices (though hopefully not all at the same time). The 1890s brought the first hormone-based remedy in the form of Ovarin, which was made from ground-up cows' ovaries, and in the 1930s menopause officially became a 'deficiency disease', and the oestrogen medication Premarin came into the market in 1942. From this point onwards, oestrogen became the go-to solution for menopause. The remedies have clearly become more humane over the years, but the fear and misogyny remain.

The history of HRT

It needs to be acknowledged that the origins of HRT came from a pretty misogynistic place. Gynaecologist Robert A. Wilson published *Feminine Forever* in 1966.[3] In tune with the times (the contraceptive pill had been made available on the NHS only five years earlier), he sold HRT as a way of women controlling their bodies. The feminism of the time concurred to some extent, perceiving the female body as needing to be medicated to get shit done, to be more productive, maybe more like a man. Living in harmony with the menstrual cycle was not a big thing for second-wave feminists, but it's easy to forget that at the time they couldn't walk down the street without either having their arse slapped or being called a slut. Wilson directed most of the book at the men whom he presumed were paying for the medication, by effectively saying that taking oestrogen replacement therapy (ERT) would prevent their wives from becoming ugly old bats. The intention with the ERT, cruelly extracted from mares' urine, was to produce a regular menstrual cycle and plump out those pesky wrinkles and rages, but it had the tragic side effect of increased breast and endometrial cancers.

'All postmenopausal women are castrates', he wrote, cheerily describing menopause as 'living decay' and postmenopausal women as 'sexual neuters'. He offered them instead the opportunity to be beautiful, sexually active, and able to please their husbands by replacing the oestrogen their bodies had lost. Clearly, this was more about being controlled than women controlling their own bodies; Robert A. Wilson was not a fan of older women, to say the least. In fact, Wilson's book *Feminine Forever* and his research foundation were both funded by Wyeth-Ayerst, the American pharmaceutical company that manufactured Premarin, which by 1975 had become the fifth leading prescription drug in the US. There *was* opposition at the time from the medical establishment; for example, Edmund R. Novak, who wrote the textbook on gynaecology, pointed out the folly of giving 60-year-old women giant doses of a potent drug to induce continuous menstruation[4].

Thankfully, things have improved since then, and a more sophisticated approach to hormone medication makes HRT a safe option. There were health scares about HRT in 2002 after a large trial had to be halted when it showed a slightly elevated risk of breast cancer and heart disease associated with the use of HRT. At the time, many were frightened into stopping their medication. The trial was badly set up because the research was not being done on women in menopause who were suffering from difficult symptoms. Instead, it used women in their sixties who may or may not have been any experiencing symptoms at all *and* who were using outdated HRT medication. If you have arrived in menopause through surgery or medication and are unable to take enough time out to completely recover, I highly recommend you take HRT. Now. It's also recommended to take HRT to protect your heart and bone health if you arrive at early menopause (i.e. before 45) at least until the age of 51, the average age of menopause.

There is an alternative view, though. What few people seem to comment on is that low oestrogen doesn't necessarily equate to menopause symptoms. The oestrogen levels present at the end of our reproductive life are roughly similar to those of prepubescent girls, but no one is medicating them, or not yet at least. There is some correlation but that does not necessarily mean that the one causes the other. HRT is a godsend for many, for sure, but plenty of people with troubling symptoms take HRT and find themselves worse and with added complications, as we'll see in chapter 10. It's hard to have to fight your corner when you're perimenopausal and to demand better treatment from your doctor, but you absolutely have the right to insist on adequate treatment.

Racism is present in women's health, as in the rest of the medical system, and menopause is no exception. For Black and ethnic minority women using HRT, it's been shown that many had not been given full information on the use of HRT before it was prescribed in the UK.

In America too, white women are more likely to be prescribed HRT than their Black counterparts, who suffer worse symptoms for a longer time.

Time and again, conventional medical doctrine judges our bodies as faulty because we are no longer fertile, when in fact living beyond our fertile years is a triumph for us and our communities. Don't forget that the medical world is based in rigidly patriarchal practices as evidenced by these fun clitoris facts: it mysteriously disappeared from the 1948 edition of the classic reference book *Gray's Anatomy – and no one even complained,* and we had to wait until 2005 when urologist Helen O'Connell proved its true size, circulation and what happened when it got excited[5] . Even today, most medical trials are still only carried out on men, as women are 'unpredictable' (meaning cyclical) and the doses are simply scaled down for women as though we were 'small men'.[6]

PRACTICE

You might like to explore the following questions as journaling prompts, in discussions with friends, to dream into them, or as inspiration for a creative project.

- How much do you consider your menopause symptoms to be a personal failure? In what way?
- Do you feel that you are failing to 'age well'? If so, how did you come by this belief?
- You might enjoy the Clearing Meditation (see page 54) to help release any negativity about ageing.

What if, instead of defining menopause as a 'deficiency condition', I celebrated it as an initiation?

Clearing Meditation

Menstruation has energetic potential: as well as the physical shedding of the womb lining, each month we also have an opportunity to release in our inner Winter that which no longer serves us, before we start again in Spring. If you have a regular cycle, a great way to do your emotional housekeeping is to use your period to release consciously whatever issue is driving you nuts. However, as our cycles reduce or stop, we may need a bit of extra help with the emotional housework – and this is where this meditation can be handy, to do a bit of energetic inner cleaning.

GETTING READY

You can use this meditation to help you let go of anything that you feel is ripe for release – be that an emotion, behaviour, a relationship, or anything that no longer serves you and feels ripe for you to let go of now. Read through the instructions first before you get started. You'll need:

- at least half an hour to yourself
- a comfortable place to sit
- cushions and blankets so you're warm and comfy
- a candle to light
- something to represent the thing you want to let go of; a natural object can be helpful
- a journal and pen to note things down later
- some chocolate or nuts to enjoy afterwards and a drink

Creating a ritual and visualizing the release is a powerful practice. It can set magic in motion for you to surrender into Wintery release and make way for Spring. If you don't have periods any more, then doing this kind of meditation can be particularly helpful to facilitate a regular release.

Carve out the time for yourself by hanging up your 'do not disturb' sign on the door, real or virtual, put your phone into 'do not disturb' mode too by turning off your Wi-Fi and/or the notifications.

There's no wrong way to do this, the meditation here is just a guide to support you to create awareness, release, and renewal. You are fully entitled to take whatever feels right for you and to ditch the rest.

THE MEDITATION

- Get really comfy using whatever cushions and seating you need so you can relax. Take a few breaths and settle into your body. Bring to mind what it is you would like to release today. Perhaps name it out loud, or say it quietly in your mind to yourself. If you'd like to write it down, or draw it, then you can do that too. Name it as you light your candle.

- Let your eyes soften or close, become aware of the way your bum makes contact with your chair or the floor, the way your back is supported, and how you feel physically grounded and supported. While your spine extends upwards, your head resting easily on your neck, let your shoulders reach downwards, your arms and hands soft.

- Breathe in through your nose and breathe out through your mouth. You can do this a few times and there might be a sigh or a yawn – that can feel good. Coming back to your natural breath, let yourself relax on the out-breath, and soften on your in-breath. Do this a few times with no effort or strain involved.

- Bring your attention to your heart and thinking of someone or something you love, see, feel or imagine this love as a golden light in your heart. Once you've established this golden love light, breathe it down through the core of your body, sending the light of love to your pelvic bowl. On the in-breath, move the golden light from the pelvic bowl up to the heart to renew the sense of love. Continue to breathe between the pelvic bowl and the heart, creating a river of light flowing up and down. You could track the flow with your eyes, sliding your gaze between your heart and your pelvic bowl if that feels nice. See how the light is filling your pelvic bowl with each breath. Each breath into the pelvis fills it a little more. Until it is brimful of love.

- As the pelvis fills with light, acknowledge the burden you have been carrying. Name the issue, person or the thing you want to release. As you feel ready, on an out-breath, let your belly and pelvis surrender and soften, so all that you are holding can flow back into the earth. Visualize, feel or imagine the golden light washing it all away. What does not serve you can now freely leave. State clearly that it's time for it to go, saying to yourself:

  - 'I forgive you ... I let you go ... I set you free ...'

- Taking a deep breath in through your nose, breathe out through your mouth; maybe do this a few times as you visualize the light or water flowing away safely, and sinking deep into the earth, letting go of whatever has held you back. If you feel any tension or tightness around your pelvis, breathe into it as you would to ignite a flame in a hot coal, trusting that everything that is ripe will release.

- Your body knows how to do this.

- You might like to rock your pelvis and move in a way that feels good, while you keep softening and relaxing as the energy or light just flows away. Do whatever helps you release, creating softness and space in the body. Continue as long as you need to, letting any tears, laughter and emotion be freely expressed. Remember that as Winter passes with its deep release, Spring will always follow and life will return.

- As the release lessens you'll start to feel lighter. Scan your body and notice any tension or stiffness, maybe in your jaw or shoulders, your thighs or heart, and find a way to move that releases the holding, letting your breath flow to help it soften.

- Come to a place of rest now. Take a breath and sigh this out through your mouth, knowing you have released. Feel the floor beneath you, your support or chair. Coming back towards the here and now, remember where you are, the objects or creatures around you, your clothes, the colours in your space.

AFTER THE MEDITATION

If you wrote down what you wanted to let go of, you might like to burn it, safely, in the candle flame. Give a word or two of gratitude for the energy of the pelvic bowl that has allowed you to release and renew so many times in your life, in so many different ways. Now blow out your candle.

Take some time to eat, to drink, and to explore in your journal what you would like to do with the object you chose to represent the thing you've let go of. What could be appropriate? You might leave it where it is, bury it, or wrap it and keep it in a safe place, before you ease back into your life.

Don't forget to stay hydrated today and when you wee or go to the loo, you can use that to confirm the release, the flushing of it away down the u-bend. Personally I try to never let an opportunity go by to release what no longer serves me.

Go gently into your day and be interested in what emerges for you. You may find you have interesting dreams and connections arise over the following days.

You can find a link to an audio of the Clearing Meditation on page 392.

5 Menopause gives us an evolutionary edge

Three species on the planet have menopause: orca whales, gall-forming aphids, and us. If we want to understand something of the evolutionary purpose of menopause, it's interesting to look at our fellow creatures to see what they get up to beyond their fertile years.

Orca whales can live to 100 years or more; and, in 2012, ecologist Darren Croft, working near Vancouver, found that postmenopausal orcas play a leadership role in the whale pod and are particularly good at finding places to hunt salmon, a primary food source[1]. They especially take the lead when times are hard, drawing on their long knowledge of their habitat. The orca grannies also stick by their adult male offspring, who are more likely to die without them near. Having menopause halfway through their life allows older female orcas to support the pod with knowledge and vitality, ensuring the survival of future generations. Elephants, who also have long lives, do not have menopause, however; and the hypothesis is that this is because unlike orca whales, their young leave the birth group to find new communities[2], so the best bet for the species is to keep on reproducing, though less often as they age.

Let us venture to a Japanese witch-hazel copse to find the *Nipponaphis monzeni*, the gall-forming aphid. Once their reproductive years have passed, the wingless female aphids turn into soldiers on a suicide mission. When a hungry ladybird wanders by looking for lunch, the postmenopausal soldiers of the colony squirt waxy glue bombs at the invader and they die slowly together. Again, the older female supports the health of the wider community.[3]

Fast forward to the Extinction Rebellion demonstrations of the last few years or any protest across the world, and you'll find sparkly-eyed, bad-ass Second Springers protecting their communities and our planet with their own glue bombs. One of the gifts that Second Spring delivers is the capacity to see through the bullshit to act in the interests of the community as a whole. As activist and herbalist Edwina Staniforth told me, postmenopausal women know how to 'stamp their feet and say NO!'. Just like the orcas and the gall-forming aphids.

PRACTICE

- Use the Clearing Meditation on page 54, to release any negative beliefs you hold about menopause.
- Reflect on the big issues that touch your community: where do your passions lie?

I have evolved to blossom in my Second Spring.

6 You can prepare for the perimenopause

If you have a menstrual cycle it offers an excellent way to prepare for menopause, because the Seasons are present through your menstrual month. The premenstrual phase is Autumnal, and has a lot in common with your perimenopause which is a more extended Life Autumn. If you can chart this part of your cycle, noticing what is challenging and how to care for yourself, you will be building a repertoire of resources to support you as perimenopause arrives.

INNER SEASONS OF MENSTRUATION
Each season represents part of your menstrual month

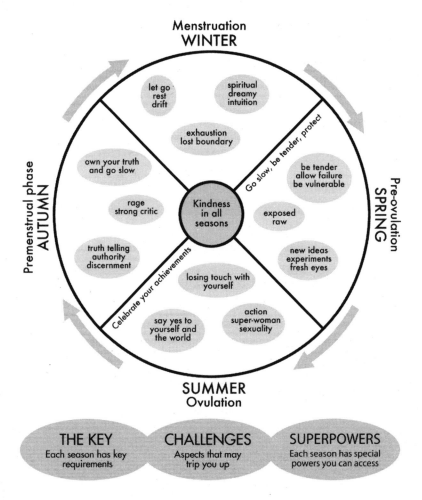

The menstrual Seasons
(created in collaboration with Leora Leboff)

I have charted my cycle for different reasons at different times in my life. In my twenties, I just wanted to know when my period was due; in my late thirties, I twice wanted to conceive; then after that I definitely didn't want to conceive. Then I forgot all about it until I was in my forties and perimenopausal and wanted to prove to myself that I was not going mad. At this uncertain time, when I trudged through endless cycles of Autumnal weariness, noting my flow and feelings every day became an anchor. A grounding cord from which I could safely regard the larger sweep of the changes that were happening within me.

'CHARTING HAS ALSO BEEN TRANSFORMATIVE. IT'S BROUGHT ME HOME TO A HOME I NEVER KNEW I HAD. I LOVE THE AUTUMNAL AND WINTER TIMES, AND THIS MAKES ME LESS FEAR-FUL ABOUT PERIMENOPAUSE AND MENOPAUSE. IT'S ALSO HELPED ME CLARIFY MY NEEDS AND MY SELF-CARE SO I FEEL PREPARED.'

Nia

The practice of menstrual cycle awareness is deceptively simple: just record your energy levels and feelings each day. That's it! Over time, in the fullness of your menstruating years, you'll start to enjoy the pattern of the Seasons as they unfold through your menstrual month: the tenderness of Spring merging into the fullness of Summer, then the Autumnal journey back into yourself before the quiet Winter of your period. It is an awesome preparation for Separation's arrival, because it develops a trust in our bodies and understanding of the ebb and flow of our energy.

Why would you chart when your cycle is completely haywire, and you cannot predict when you're going to be feeling a particular way? Even if you've never charted before you arrived in perimenopause, it is an excellent time to start. Though your menstrual Seasons may not behave in a sequential order, the daily mapping has a number of benefits:

- It validates your experience of what you are feeling: by noting your various emotions in a day, you can own your feelings. It also helps you to own your range of expression and own the darker parts of yourself.
- It helps you to track cause and effect: by charting physical and psychological problems and events you can track things such as how stress affects you, if any dietary changes are having an effect, or what interrupts your sleep.
- It uses the awesome power of naming: by recognizing 'I am in Surrender today', or Spring, or what-have-you, it bypasses a lot of what gets in the way of us being kind to ourselves. For example, I might feel really sluggish and sad and want to stay under the duvet: I could drag myself out and force myself to complete my to-do list; or I could recognize this as Winter and show myself Winter kindness, spending a little more time in bed and allowing myself to go slow and rest.
- Insight: it gives you a great resource when engaging with emotional processing, by adding your dreams when you wake up, for example, or seeing how your week went after a particular insight. In the longer term, you can become witness to your own process by reviewing old charts and celebrate your journey.
- Even the smallest act of self-care, like slowing down a little, will have knock-on benefits later in your cycle.

Just noticing the changes in your cycle is a mindfulness practice in itself. Over the months, you'll begin to see patterns emerging and shifting, and you'll be able to see how stress affects you differently at different times of the month. Psychologically, tracking your menstrual cycle helps us to integrate all aspects of ourselves, especially the parts that are not so easily appreciated by our nearest and dearest. It debunks the whole myth of having a universally nice, capable way of being because the 'nice, capable' part is oestrogenic.

'WHAT I LEARNED AT THE PRE-MENSTRUUM TURNED OUT TO BE INVALUABLE BECAUSE MY SUPERPOWER WAS RAGE. I LEARNED TO OBSERVE THAT AND SEE THAT IT ONLY HAPPENED FOR A BRIEF PERIOD. AND MENOPAUSE GOES ON FOR EIGHT YEARS.'

Uma Dinsmore-Tuli, activist and author of Yoni Shakti

You can use these last bleeds as a precious time to help you embrace your darker aspects too, and accept the power and depth of who you are. As you journey down your perimenopausal path, you'll probably find that your cycle develops more and more of an Autumnal flavour: the ovulatory Summers might get shorter and you may skip a few ovulations here and there. Don't be surprised if you find yourself grieving, perhaps without a particular focus, as Autumn is the natural home of grief.

But take heart: that great speaker of girls' and women's truths, the awesome Caitlin Moran has compared perimenopause to coming down off Ecstasy;[1] having been jumping around hugging everyone and being happy in your Life Summer, you are now out of forgiveness for the things that other people do and have discovered your actual personality. In short, Life Autumn, your perimenopause, brings you home to yourself. It can be a great shock but you can lessen it by practising charting during your menstruating years.

Contemplating perimenopause can sometimes feel overwhelming, especially when there is lots of advice out there. My number one top tip to prepare for the adventures ahead is to slow down and rest when you have your period.

PRACTICE

On a chart or app consider noting:

- How I'm feeling.
- Any pain.
- Sleep.
- Physical problems.
- Energy levels.
- Dietary changes.
- Digestive problems.
- Dreams.
- Events like travel.
- Stressful situations.
- Periods.
- Ovulation.
- Cervical mucus consistency.
- What Inner Seasons are present for me?
- What menopause phases do I most identify with?
- Complementary therapy appointments.
- Supplements taken.

MENSTRUAL CYCLE CHART

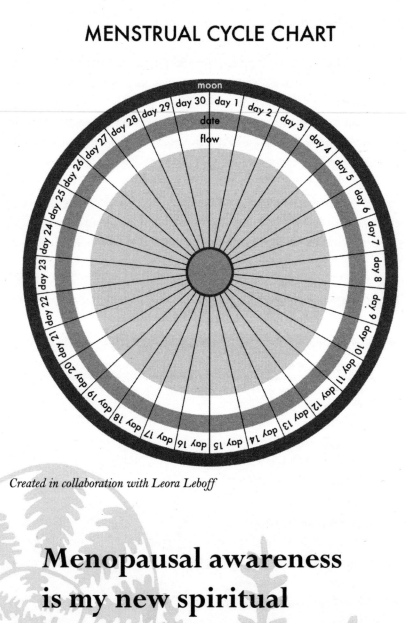

moon

day 30 | day 1 | day 2 | day 3 | day 4 | day 5 | day 6 | day 7 | day 8 | day 9 | day 10 | day 11 | day 12 | day 13 | day 14 | day 15 | day 16 | day 17 | day 18 | day 19 | day 20 | day 21 | day 22 | day 23 | day 24 | day 25 | day 26 | day 27 | day 28 | day 29

date

flow

Created in collaboration with Leora Leboff

Menopausal awareness is my new spiritual practice.

7 Honour the blood and tears

Ms Perfectly Average will have around 444 menstrual cycles in her lifetime. Think about it: 444 Inner Autumns and Winters followed by Inner Springs and Summers. No wonder it's such a loss when our cycle goes, because even when it brings us challenges we know what to expect. There's a predictable rhythm, which, even if we hate it, gives us inner pacing and teaches us how we are cyclical beings. Consciously or not, we are constantly moving outwards to show ourselves to the world in our menstrual Springs and Summers, before coming back inward to tend to our inner lives in Autumn and Winter. Ultimately, this rhythm connects us deeply to the earth.

'I KNEW MENOPAUSE WAS ON THE HORIZON BECAUSE MY CENTRE OF BALANCE SHIFTED.'

'Patricia'

To move into menopause, we must honour and commemorate the periods we've had and the lessons our cycles have taught us before we can let this part of our lives go. Have a party, buy flowers, wear a red dress, wear your 444 badge with pride; you've earned it. It's never too late to do this either: a retrospective celebration of your menstruating years can be just as meaningful.

PRACTICE

Find ways of celebrating your menstruating life. Ideas might include:

- Creating a ritual alone or with friends.
- Adding up how many periods you've had in your life.
- Finding a poem or song that reflects your bleeding years.
- Express yourself creatively through painting, dancing, singing, or crafting.
- Buying a special piece of jewellery, a garment or artwork.

I have earned my place at the feast.

8 Suicide

There is a hidden mental health crisis that affects women in midlife. Headlines about suicide are usually concerned with the risks for young and middle-aged men and it's true that rates are three times higher for men, but for women, the highest suicide rate is between the ages of 45 to 49 years and it's been rising exponentially over time; in the US, suicide remains among the top 10 leading causes of death for these years[1].

The way we choose to present ourselves to the outside world with our shiny coping persona is always a lie (good to remember when you're scrolling through your social media) but at menopause it's a BIG FAT

DANGEROUS lie. In the public sphere, witty handbag designer Kate Spade, film producer Jill Messick, and journalist Sally Brampton all took their lives and British media personality Carol Vorderman went public about having suicidal thoughts, all prompting 'Menopause drove me to suicide' headlines.

But is this menopause killing them? Kathryn Abel, Professor of Psychological Medicine at the Centre for Women's Mental Health at the University of Manchester, says we can put it down to 'lifestyle'. This means the classic sandwich of having kids later (with the likelihood of depleting fertility treatments and miscarriage) with caring for elderly parents, served up with a big dollop of financial pressure, all pushing women close to breakdown when menopause years bring more sensitivity. She says:

The feeling of failing is a very typical way women resolve their distress. They internalize it and take on the guilt. But the causes don't matter – the solutions do. Women have to recognize when they need help, such as inability to sleep, a restless mind, lack of concentration and not enjoying things you'd normally enjoy. [2]

The dissonance between the outer mask and our inner feelings – that we're failing, that we're useless, trapped, not strong enough and should be able to cope and look perfect doing it – are killing us. The rigid feminine identity of endless caregiver, coupled with life circumstances, sometimes mean that it is impossible to release the roles that cause breakdown and risk suicide. Poverty, racial and gender discrimination, abuse, loneliness, trauma, as well as a history of poor mental health, are all factors that when coupled with the shifting hormones in perimenopause can become a serious risk.

Studies on the risk of suicide and self-harming behaviour in younger women show that there is greater risk in the premenstrual phase, i.e. in the Autumn of the menstrual cycle, mirroring the elevated risk during Life Autumn, perimenopause. [3] From a Seasonal perspective, we understand that there is no respect given for the Autumn/Winter side of the cycle. The requirements for a happy Autumn and Winter – spaciousness, quiet, inner focus, reflection, and dreaming – are not available to most of us. If we were allowed to withdraw in our Autumn and Winter and take our foot off the gas, this would give us the space we need to restore and heal. Meanwhile, the pressure of our inner needs in the face of societal and financial demands raises the risk of breakdown, self-harm, and suicide.

Unfortunately, because there is so little research around menopause and mental health, it's not yet possible to understand exactly what is happening – and there are as many studies show *no* worsening in mental health as there are that do – but there's no doubt that the negativity around ageing and menopause contributes to feelings of hopelessness.

There is a list of specialist helplines in the Resources on page 397.

It's OK to ask for help.

If You Feel Suicidal

- Try to focus on getting through this hour, rather than thinking about the future.
- Talk to someone you trust or a helpline about how you are feeling; it doesn't matter if you feel you don't deserve help or that it won't make a difference.
- Contact a health professional like your doctor or community mental health team.
- Try to do activities that take your mind off what you're thinking.
- If you are in danger call 999 or go to A&E.

IF YOU ARE WORRIED ABOUT SOMEONE

Even a friendly smile and a warm chat can let them know they are cared for and not alone. Don't be afraid to ask them directly if they have suicidal thoughts; it's not true that talking about it might make it more likely.

If they have a plan, the intention and the means to kill themselves, call 999.

Listen non-judgementally and encourage them to talk about what they're feeling and thinking.

Reassure them that these thoughts are common, they don't have to act on them, and that suicidal thoughts are often associated with a treatable mental illness[1].

Encourage them to get support from a trusted loved one or professional.

Encourage them to think about what self-help has worked for them in the past, and which people and/or communities were helpful.

Don't forget to find some self-help for yourself afterwards, talking through what happened with a trusted friend or professional.

9 Symptoms vary by culture

According to the available research, American Black women have the worst menopause symptoms[1], but, as yet, the necessary research hasn't been done to explain why this is so. Looking across the global experience, there's significant variation according to culture, diet, lifestyle, and how ageing is regarded – and this shows us that *there is no fixed, biological inevitability that menopause will be vile.* However, stress – especially in the form of racial trauma – is certainly playing its part[2].

In the UK, although 13.8 per cent of the population are from an ethnic minority background, there's been a pathetic amount of research into the experience of menopause in Black and ethnic minority communities, despite evidence from the US that menopause arrives earlier, lasts longer, and the physiological symptoms are more severe for Black women. With a wide variation in symptoms in the UK, joint and muscle aches being common in Indian and Pakistani women, for example, there's great potential for misdiagnosis and mistreatment even without a language barrier[3]. On the website MegsMenopause.com, Dr Nighat Arif explains:

> *Women have come to believe that the menopause is a 'white, middle class' problem or a 'Western phenomenon'. In Punjabi/Urdu there is no direct translation for the word 'menopause'. Women only partially understand it; referring to that point in life where their hormones change as 'old age' or 'no longer able to bear children', or simply 'periods have stopped'.*[4]

This shameful situation has been taken up by Second Spring designer and podcaster Karen Arthur from her platform Menopause Whilst Black, where she gathers stories of Black British women's experience of menopause to raise visibility of Black menopause and help them better navigate support systems. In an interview with *Vogue* magazine, she says:

I was thinking, what are my other Black menopausal women doing, and how are they coping with their symptoms? How are they dealing with seeing people who look like our sons, our brothers, our relatives, our daughters, Breonna Taylor, Ahmaud Arbery, and so many others [being killed]? How are they coping with that on top of menopausal symptoms? On top of Covid? Menopause is a lot in itself. Being a Black person in a white supremacist society is a lot. [5]

Given how stress disrupts the endocrine system, imagine how long-term racial trauma across many generations is going to affect a menopausal body. On top of this, the constant re-traumatization and defence against micro-aggressions that women of colour have to contend with on a daily basis negatively impacts their endocrine systems. In a feature for *Good Housekeeping* magazine, journalist Paula Akpan argues:

Menopause is yet another arena of gross medical racism where race and cultural background aren't properly taken into consideration. [6]

Coming into menopause under these circumstances, especially when you've had to work twice as hard as a white woman to get where you are, is going to be tough. Added to which, the only UK research, on a very small number of women of colour, showed that they did not get access to sufficient information about treatment. Dr Nitu Bajekal, gynaecologist, states:

My own clinical experience, spanning 35 years as a specialist in Obstetrics and Gynaecology with an interest in menopause, and seeing patients from all backgrounds and races in my clinics, is that Black and Asian women are less likely to seek medical help or want hormone replacement. [7]

There's a fair bit of research into menopause in Japan, where only about 25 per cent of women experience hot flushes, as opposed to 75 per cent in the UK, although some research indicated that flushes existed but weren't talked about. Instead, women expect to have stiff shoulders, lumbago and feel chilly during their transition.[8] Having a health tradition of disease prevention rather than cure means diet, exercise, and a more positive attitude towards ageing all play a part in there being fewer cases of osteoporosis, breast cancer, and high blood pressure than in the West. Menopause in Japan is understood to be a sensitive time of renewal rather than ovarian depletion or failure.[9,10,11,12,]

There are other cultures too where menopause isn't feared: Mayan women, the Maori of New Zealand, and the Iroquois Indians looked forward to menopause when they became spiritual leaders in their communities.[13,14,15] In cultures where women have had traditionally low status, as in India, menopause can bring more freedom to go out and about in the world, which would have been forbidden in their earlier years.[16,17]

Symptoms vary by economic status and interestingly it's not always as you'd expect. In the US and Europe, the poorest women suffer most, but in Pakistan it's the wealthy that complain about more symptoms. In general, it seems in cultures and countries where there is a matriarchal system, menopause symptoms are less severe.[18] Whether the differences can be nailed down to stress, beliefs, diet, lifestyle or culture is not clear, but for sure, you can see that there is no *inevitable* decline, symptom or consequence of menopause. As menstrual shame is being dismantled bit by bit, there is hope that for my daughter's generation, when they arrive at menopause, there will be celebration rather than medication awaiting them.

David Sturdee, whose study showed that British women have the worst symptoms, has said that:

This study tells us as much about the quality of life of older women as it does about the clinical signs of aging … it's also clear that these countries [where symptoms are less severe] tend to be matriarchal societies where older women are revered for their wisdom.[19]

David Sturdee is president of the International Menopause Society, right in the heart of the establishment, saying that he has found in his research, that there are fewer menopause symptoms in societies that value women.

This is not Kate's 'woo-woo' take on the subject: this is proper science backed by studies that show how negative expectations of menopause can become a self-fulfilling prophecy. Living in a patriarchal society makes us more tired, irritable, depressed, achy, hot, sleepless, and gives us a headache.[20,21] But you knew that already.

PRACTICE

You might like to explore these questions as journaling prompts or discussions with friends, to dream into them, or as inspiration for a creative project. You get to choose how you define menopause.

- What cultural beliefs do you hold about menopause? Do they work for you?
- What do older female relatives say about their experience?
- Use the Clearing Meditation on page 54 to help clear unwanted beliefs.
- If you would prefer to find a different way of looking at this time of life, what would that look like?
- Use the Self-Care Abdominal Massage (see pages 74–76) with the intention of affirming a positive menopause experience.

I had the power all the time.

Self-Care Abdominal Massage

Created by herbalist Rosita Arvigo[1], the gentle practice of self-care abdominal massage can make a dramatic difference to how much you can love yourself. You can't get this wrong if it feels good! You're also likely to see an improvement in physical symptoms such as:

- period pain
- digestive issues
- a great variety of 'interesting' menopause issues

WHY DOES IT WORK?
Massaging your belly will help by:

- improving circulation to your womb and digestive organs
- releasing tension in the tissues and fascia
- reducing scar tissue
- dissolving emotional blocks
- helping to realign your womb
- soothing you by reducing cortisol and increasing oxytocin

WHEN TO DO IT
- Before you go to sleep.
- Three times a week for a month and track the changes.
- Start the day after your period finishes.
- Continue till a few days before you start your next period.

WHEN NOT TO DO IT
- a few days before, during or immediately after your period
- if you have an IUD or coil of any kind
- if you think you might be pregnant
- if you have an infection
- if you're taking pain killers which might mask any pain

GUIDELINES
- For your massage you'll need some oil, body lotion or massage balm, a warm room, a couple of pillows and 15 minutes to yourself.
- Be gentle with yourself, breathe, use slow strokes and make sure it feels good.
- Pressing your shoulder blades into your support will help to release tension.

WHAT TO DO

Lie on your back and get comfy by putting a pillow under your knees.

Place your hands on your belly between your belly button and pubic bone and take long, slow breaths into your abdomen until you feel relaxed.

If you are using a mantra, bring it to mind and send it through your hands, and into your belly. If you have no particular mantra, send a smile down to your belly and notice how it responds.

Using your oil or lotion, make slow circles in a clockwise direction around the periphery of your belly. From hipbone to hipbone, up the sides, under the rib cage and down again. This is the direction that your digestion flows through your colon. Keep your touch light at first and your hands soft on your belly. Deepen your touch to see what feels good.

Next, work between your hipbones. Using the pads of your middle three fingers, one hand on top of the other, start just by the left hipbone, and make spiralling circles across, just above your pubic bone, over to the right hipbone. Then spiral in circles back across the pubic bone to the left. Repeat at a pleasurable depth as often as feels good. You are massaging over your womb. Giving her gentle attention helps the flow of blood and lymph, the nerve impulses and the flow of energy.

Very gently, feel down your breast bone to the soft place just where it ends at a spot called the xiphoid process. Very softly, rest the tips of your middle three fingers of your non-dominant hand here. It's a really tender place, which can hold a lot of charge, so just resting your fingers here might be enough. If you want more, massage this space very gently. Breathe. Enjoy your out-breath.

Place your hands just underneath your ribcage, the heels of your hands on each side, your middle fingers resting on or just below the xiphoid process. With the pressure in the heels of your hands, on an out-breath, sweep diagonally down from ribs to belly button, inviting your diaphragm to release. Repeat this a couple of times.

Now rest the heels of your hands on your waist at the sides of the body. And on an out-breath, strongly stroke the heels of your hands towards your belly button. Repeating this again, as often and as deep as you like.

Finally, place your hands over your womb space or womb and enjoy the new energy you have created. Notice the sensations. Notice if you feel different to when you started.

If you are using a mantra today, send that down, once again, into your belly. If you weren't using a mantra, send another big smile down into your belly and womb.

KEEP ON BEING GENTLE WITH YOURSELF

Don't forget to drink lots of water and to notice what happens with your symptoms. Stay curious about what is happening. Your womb may have a clear out with a heavier period than usual. You might have some interesting poo, or feel sore if you are new to this practice.

There may also be an emotional release so be gentle and kind to yourself if you find that you're emotional. Working with your body in this deep, yet respectful way is deeply healing.

If you wish, you can access a video of how to do the Self-Care Abdominal Massage at my website: katecodrington.co.uk

10 When to use HRT

This book is all about how to use your menopause for growth and HRT can definitely be part of that picture. You might have decided on a natural route but have been slayed by life circumstances or overwhelmed by symptoms. Conversely, you might be firmly attached to a medical approach but want to understand your psychological transition better. All paths are valid. HRT, like all women's health, can be a highly charged area with people defending their positions with the tenacity of tigers, but there's no right way to do this, no prize for muscling through misery or sailing through it all with serenity. There's only our own process and our kindness towards ourselves, which is as unique as we are.

'I HAD SEVERE PANIC ATTACKS WHICH HAVE RESULTED IN ME NOT BEING ABLE TO DRIVE ON THE MOTORWAY. I THINK THIS WAS BROUGHT ON BY NOT ALLOWING MYSELF THE TIME AND SPACE TO GRIEVE PROPERLY FOR MY DAD. EXPERIENCING HIGH LEVELS OF ANXIETY, I TRIED ANTI-DEPRESSANTS WHICH JUST MADE ME FEEL NUMB, AND I PUFFED UP LIKE A BALLOON. I RESEARCHED HRT AND IT DEFINITELY MADE A BIG DIFFERENCE, ALONG WITH GETTING HYPNOTHERAPY AND GIVING MYSELF MORE SPACE. WITHIN WEEKS MY SYMPTOMS REDUCED AND I FELT SO MUCH BETTER. I NO LONGER HAVE ANY JOINT PAIN, BRAIN FOG IS MINIMAL, ANXIETY IS SIGNIFICANTLY REDUCED.'

'Heather'

Benefits

Taking HRT is safe these days: most are 'bioidentical', meaning that they are plant based and structurally identical to your own hormones. However, HRT is not a one-size-fits-all prescription; it needs tailoring to your specific hormone balance and different brands are better at addressing different symptoms. You may well need to try some of the many different doses and/or brands to find what works for you. This can take time, so it's worth being persistent and returning to your doctor to work out a new solution together if you need to.

If you have a womb, you will need to take progesterone alongside the oestrogen to prevent the lining of the womb from building up, which can increase the risk of endometrial cancer. If you still have periods, the HRT will enable you to continue your monthly cycle and this HRT, known as 'sequential combined therapy', is usually taken for a year or so. If you have a hormonal coil that releases progesterone, you can just add in the oestrogen through a patch or gel. If it's been a year or more since your last period, then your HRT will be the kind where you don't have a period, known as 'continuous combined therapy'. If you don't have a womb, you will be given oestrogen-only HRT. If your libido is still low after taking HRT, then you could explore testosterone supplementation. Because most of the testosterone is made in the ovaries, if you've had them removed, it's likely your T levels (testosterone levels) will be low. With any degree of vaginal atrophy, topical oestrogen cream carries little risks and should help to manage symptoms (see chapter 48), and lubricants can be helpful.[1]

HRT has also been shown to reduce the risk of cardiovascular disease. It can prevent and reverse bone loss while you are taking it, but bone loss will resume once you stop taking HRT.[2] The jury is out on its effects on Alzheimer's, with studies going both ways.[3, 4]

Tania Elfersy, a transformative coach who guides women to natural relief for their menopause symptoms, says:

*I wouldn't call HRT a solution, but it can be part of a woman's journey.
Sometimes a woman will benefit from 'turning the volume down' on her
symptoms so that she can better cope with life. From that quieter space,
she'll be able to listen to her body, allowing the healing to begin.*

Risks

HRT is not recommended if you have problems with your liver, high
blood pressure, a thickening of the lining of the womb, thrombosis,
oestrogen-sensitive cancers or breast cancer. Common side effects of
HRT can include vaginal bleeding or spotting, sore breasts, nausea, or
cramping in your legs. Patches seem to be the favoured delivery method,
although just occasionally, people report skin irritation, so different brands
may suit your skin better.

Those with a history of hormonal cancers should be aware that there
is a small increase in the risk of breast and endometrial cancer from using
particular kinds of combined HRT *if you are over 51.*[5] This only continues
for as long as you are taking the HRT and no increased risk of early death
has been shown. Taking body-identical progesterone does not appear to
be associated with an increased risk of breast cancer for the first five years
of taking it. This has been equated to the same as having one glass of
wine a day, but less than the risk of drinking two glasses, or the same as
being overweight or not exercising much. Numerous studies have shown
that women who take oestrogen-only HRT do not have a higher risk of
breast cancer. Some studies have even shown these women have a lower
risk of breast cancer.[6]

Women who take some HRT tablets have a slightly higher risk of
developing a clot in their veins or having a stroke, especially if you have
other risk factors. Using oestrogen gel or patches instead of tablets
eliminates the risk[7] . A history of migraine, diabetes or liver disease will
also indicate (i.e. make advisable) the use of patches or gel.

'I FELT LIKE MYSELF AGAIN.'

'Penny'

The benefits of HRT can usually be felt within two weeks, with moodiness, sleep and flushes improving. A lifesaver for sure, as there are many stories of women alive today who considered taking their own life before they took HRT.[8] I'd hazard a guess that if women's cycles were respected and the need for a quiet retreat in Autumn and Winter were widely understood, this would not be so common.

I'd like to examine the phrase 'I feel like myself again'. As menopause is an agent of transformation, our 'old self' is required to open and be released for the possibilities of Second Spring to emerge. The relief of 'feeling like ourselves' is palpable, we're on solid ground here, but on this solid ground, perhaps we lose the possibilities for growth.

I feel it's a bit like taking the pill, it sort of puts stuff on hold. those it suits seem to stay in that pre-menopausal place, i feel, of having lots of yang energy, doing more and not quietening or going inwards.
Mary Hurley, women's health acupuncturist

It's very human to want to fix the pain and go back to normal. Of course we'd love a magic pill, but menopause is like the caterpillar's journey. It requires a strong cocoon in the form of boundaries and support. We're going to spend quite a lot of time inside it, being mush. We wish it was quick and less messy, but it's not *and* it takes time. If we try to break out of the cocoon too early, it makes us too vulnerable, but if we can lean into our support, trusting that we are being held by the process of menopause, we can emerge a different creature; a better version of ourselves. Unless you embark on a healing journey through therapy or menstrual cycle awareness, for example, taking HRT will make you a very competent caterpillar, but what if you miss out on being a butterfly?

How long?

How long you take HRT is a personal decision. There's a myth that if you stop taking HRT, then you will automatically be engulfed by the evil mother of all menopauses, but actually, once you stop taking HRT, you'll have whatever symptoms would have been there without medication anyway. Menopause invites you to slow down and look inwards, and taking HRT can allow you to bypass this. The oestrogen will enable you to focus and be active in the outside world, so when you stop taking HRT, unless you significantly slow down or take a menopause gap (see chapter 57), you will be in the realm of collapse. Under the guidance of your doctor, you can safely take HRT for as long as you need to[9]. From my experience of clients, I still advise those on HRT to slow down, and take that inward, reflective time for themselves so they can make their transition with minimal discomfort.

Different types

You can use HRT skin patches or gel, and there are many different brands and preparations[10]. The most commonly prescribed in the UK is estradiol, a 'bioidentical' oestrogen made from yams that has the same molecular structure as the oestrogen that declines in your body. Rarely prescribed now, the old-style HRT made from pregnant mares' urine had so many associated side effects, it's been largely phased out. Another product derived from the wonderful yam is micronized progesterone, which has the same molecular structure as your body's own progesterone, so has fewer side effects.

Bespoke HRT

It is possible to obtain a bespoke prescription, known as compounded hormones or BHRT. These will be custom-made to match your specific hormone picture, but it's worth checking that what you are being offered has been officially approved, because tinkering around with your hormone balance is a delicate business and you can end up with some nasty side effects. So far, there's no evidence to show that compounded HRT is safer or better than 'bioidentical' options, so if you decide to take the former route, it's best to check out your menopause expert's credentials.

Making your mind up

Sadly, many doctors receive minimal training in menopause and some people have difficulty obtaining HRT, but it is worth persisting to advocate for the good care you need. We live complex lives, with complex demands made of us. Each of us will have different vulnerabilities, risk factors, and needs. Making your mind up takes time, a well-informed doctor or menopause specialist, and an awareness of the bigger picture in your life.

PRACTICE

People often ask me whether taking HRT will stop them from making the psychological transition. My observation is that as it 'turns down the volume' on the symptoms, it might turn down the volume on the wisdom or conversely help you attune more to your cycle. Whether you take HRT or not, you will *still* need to:

- Manage stress.
- Cut the crap food.
- Do your emotional work.
- Cut the crap beliefs.
- Rest more than you feel is reasonable.

Slow down, rest, and nourish yourself.

11 What to ask your doctor

Consulting doctors can be stressful at the best of times, but when you're in the mush stage of becoming a butterfly, it can be especially hard. I've made a list of questions for you to take with you to an appointment with your doctor so you can work out your best possible treatment together. Unfortunately, not all doctors are up to speed with the latest guidelines and, according to Nuffield research, a quarter of those who visited a doctor say the possibility of the symptoms being menopause-related was missed.[1]

Many of us are still being prescribed SSRIs or antidepressants instead of HRT, which is against the current best practice guidelines.[2] Clearly there is a fair bit of education to be had by many general practitioners in the UK, but there are specialists in gynaecological health to be found in most practices, so it's worth asking when you book your appointment. If you're lucky, there may even be a menopause specialist.

Preparing for your appointment

- Ask for a longer appointment; the standard 10 minutes probably won't be enough.
- If you are following the practice outlined in chapter 6, you'll already be charting your symptoms, so you can create a record of what you've been experiencing, the duration and an indication of severity. This should include your periods too if you have them.
- Write a list of all the medication, herbs, and supplements you're taking, the doses and frequency.
- Write a list of any life stressors or trauma from the last year, even if you feel you're over them.
- Write a list of conditions that you have experienced personally and in your family history, especially if there's heart disease, osteoporosis, cancer, diabetes etc.
- Print off a copy of the NICE guidelines to take with you.[3]

What to ask

Not all of the following questions may be appropriate for you, so use this list as a starting point and choose those appear most appropriate for your personal circumstances.

1. Could my symptoms be caused by something other than menopause?
2. Could I be pregnant?
3. What about contraception – what's the best option for me?
4. What tests can you run to assess my hormone balance?
5. What other tests are available elsewhere that might be helpful?
6. Is there a menopause specialist you can refer me to?
7. What herbs and/or supplements would you recommend?
8. Are there any non-hormonal treatments that might help?
9. What would the benefits of HRT be for me?
10. What are the risks of HRT for me?
11. What are the risks of not taking HRT?
12. What are the side effects of HRT?
13. For how long is it safe for me to take it?
14. What kind of HRT would you recommend?
15. What are the advantages and disadvantages of using patches, cream or tablets?
16. What are my risks for breast cancer, heart disease and osteoporosis?
17. Should I get screening for osteoporosis, cancer or heart disease?
18. Would HRT interact with any of the other herbs, supplements and medication I am taking?
19. What's the lowest dose I could start with?
20. How do you work out the right dose for me?
21. What can I do about my libido?
22. Do you recommend testosterone supplementation?
23. I have pain in my vulva and/or vagina: what treatment will help with this?
24. Can you recommend an oestrogen cream?
25. How frequently should I come back for check-ups?
26. When should I stop taking HRT?
27. What's the protocol for stopping taking HRT?

I am fully entitled to get answers to my questions and choose the treatment I prefer.

12 Complementary allies

I am often asked what kind of complementary therapy I would recommend for this or that symptom, but as a long-time therapy junkie, it's been my experience that it's not the modality but the relationship with the therapist that is the key to success. Numerous studies[1][2] have shown that it's a positive relationship and rapport with your therapist that determines positive outcomes. If you are employing professional support, and you don't have a place of safety and trust, no healing can happen, no matter what modality they use. Your body has a natural impulse to move towards healing and it only requires the right environment to allow this to happen; you need to feel heard and witnessed to have your experience validated. To be 'held', meaning that your therapist makes safe boundaries for you so you can soften and release without fear of judgement, allows emotional cycles to complete themselves.

Perverse as it seems, the more we try to change, the more stuck we become. This was named 'the paradoxical theory of change' by the founder of Gestalt Psychotherapy, Fritz Perls.[1] He said that the therapist must reject the role of 'changer' because this implies that the client is 'not OK'. Healing happens when we accept 'what is', like in the phase of Surrender, and this is a vital requirement when you're looking for a therapist. Menopause is delivering you into *your* authority and you do not need someone who pathologizes or tries to fix you into a better version of yourself; you are OK just as you are. You're a beautiful human, not a fixer-upper bought at a bargain price to make a fat profit.

Try to find a personal recommendation where you can. Chat to your therapist by phone or Zoom to get a feel for what they're like and notice your body's response. It's an expensive business, so give yourself time and space to see if you'd feel safe with them before you book. You are the authority on you and just because a therapist has a shiny website and a long waiting list, it doesn't necessarily mean they'll be a great match.

There is precious little research, and so much variation in practice and personal therapy styles and integrations, that it's impossible to tell in advance which complementary therapies are going to work for you and sort out your issues. Sometimes you'll see an immediate improvement, sometimes not. Sometimes it works for a long time, sometimes it seems to stop working after a while. The best complementary therapies will ease the physical challenges, while empowering you to make better choices in your life. Here are some suggestions to consider:

Abdominal massage: also known as womb or abdominal-sacral massage, it literally addresses the core issues of being in a female body, both physical and psychological. Heavenly. (See pages 74–76 for information on how to do this for yourself.)

Acupuncture: Chinese medicine has been practised for thousands of years and though the theory can be pretty impenetrable, it works well to support the menopausal transition.

Biodynamic: touch-based therapy focused on completing emotional cycles and being with what is.

Counselling/psychotherapy: to work on specific issues via Zoom or face-to-face, there's a talking therapy to suit every taste.

Functional medicine: figures out how and why illness occurs and restores health by addressing root causes.

Medical herbalist: Great for menopause, herbalists combine an encyclopaedic medical knowledge with ancient understanding of herbs.

Menstruality Medicine Circle facilitation: if you want to dive deeper into your Inner Seasons and the phases to find your way forward, there are 1-2-1 and group sessions available. (See also chapter 16 and the Resources section.)

Shiatsu: all the heft of Chinese medicine but using touch instead of needles.

Yoga nidra: the gentle guided meditation practice anyone can do. 1-2-1 sessions can offer bespoke nidras (or meditations) for your situation, or there are group classes you can join, or audios to download from my website (see Resources, page 392).

Access allies that support your authority.

13 Multi-gendered pause

Menopause doesn't only happen to cis women. It happens to trans men, to non-binary, and intersex folk too. We've touched on how sharing experiences normalizes our difficulties and how our perceived value affects symptoms, so what about the experience of people who do not identify as cis women? Where does menopause, or a menopause-like transition occur if you were assigned female at birth but don't identify as a woman?

For a trans guy, whatever age you start taking testosterone, or when adjusting the dosage, or if you have a hysterectomy and have ovaries removed, you will experience menopause transition. Some non-binary, genderfluid, agender, bi+ gender, and other related gender people who have a womb and ovaries, and who are not taking hormones, will also have a menopause. Trans women will also have a mini-menopause when they reduce the oestrogen they're taking, before bottom surgery.

While fashion brands are moving towards non-gendered marketing, when you Google menopause, nearly every image has a grey-haired, white woman with gorgeous cheekbones looking worried and wearing hot pink, fanning herself. If I, as a cis white woman, can't identify with these images, then how is it for the rainbow of gender non-conforming folk? If you don't see yourself represented and there are not places to share your experience and get support, you are doubly marginalized.

'I WOULDN'T FEEL SAFE TO EXPRESS
MYSELF IN A GENDERED "WOMEN ONLY
SPACE", IT RISKS INVASIVE INTERROGATION
ABOUT MY GENDER IDENTITY OR BEING
REJECTED. BECAUSE OF THE "FUCK IT"
ASPECT OF MENOPAUSE, I WON'T PUT
UP WITH IT. I'VE FINISHED SQUASHING
MYSELF INTO OTHER PEOPLE'S
ACCEPTABLE NORMALITIES.'

Samantha, non-binary and genderfluid

As I see menopause as primarily a transformational process, I want to open up more conversations about how this manifests for trans men and women and non-binary people in a nuanced way, without the almighty charge that this discussion can have. I was really curious about menopause experiences outside the visible range to see what was going on and how the transformation played out. But doing the research put me in a highly dodgy position: many people before me have marched into the trans and non-binary communities, sucked up their tender stories, and then used them to elevate their own profile, leaving the communities beached. Most people I approached wouldn't talk to me; they had likely learned to be wary the hard way. All the research and stories in this chapter and elsewhere were given in full knowledge that I was writing this book. I have been lucky, though, in connecting with some beautiful souls who were generous enough to offer their experiences as a gift, to expand the awareness of the transformational possibilities menopause might hold.

For men of trans experience, taking testosterone, hormone blockers or having a hysterectomy will create a menopause-type experience as their oestrogen is subsumed or ceases. Many, but not all, feel forced to be ultra-male in ways that cis men don't have to be and so embracing menstruation or menopause can be a difficult thing for outsiders to understand. Activist @kennyethanjones speaks eloquently about how he embraces his periods, for example.

Though not thinking about it in terms of menopause, because that's something that 'happens to cis women', arriving at his longed-for gender transition, G. McGregor, man of trans experience, described the relief:

I felt slowly, gently, my new dominant hormone took its deserved place in my body as if it were coming home and the no longer dominant hormone gracefully took a backseat, knowing it wasn't needed anymore. I essentially shed this vessel that had known all along it wasn't the right fit. I even found myself saying 'goodbye my old friend'; I was embodying the real me.

This beautiful, nuanced explanation moved me to tears: it shows how it can be possible to accept all of who we are. It's a long way from the either/or, yes/no tick-box reduction of the mainstream narrative. Other trans men shared how, when they started taking testosterone, it felt easeful and how the anxiety and body dysmorphia they had been experiencing for years seemed to magically disappear.

'THE T [TESTOSTERONE]

INSTANTLY FELT RIGHT IN MY

SYSTEM. I HAD DEBILITATING

ANXIETY ISSUES BEFORE BUT IT

CLEARED THEM UP VERY QUICKLY.'

'Angela', woman of trans experience

Undergoing the chemical or surgical treatment does create a physiological menopause and although trans men weren't particularly relating to their experience as such, they were still undergoing the transformational shift towards their true selves, shedding identities and old ways of being, just as cis women do. In their case though, it was the accumulation of years of aching to be different, of shrugging their old, unwanted selves from their shoulders. A much longed for transition.

From the generous trans women who spoke to me, having survived the arduous journey to gender reassignment, they generally seem to embrace their oestrogen with such joy and relief, that lessening the dose to create a menopause would seem frankly insane. Having worked so hard to get here, why would you ever give it up?

NO WAY IN HELL WILL THEY TAKE AWAY MY OESTROGEN, I'M PLANNING TO STAY ON IT WELL BEYOND SEVENTIES. I WASTED TOO MUCH OF MY LIFE ALREADY.

Janet, 'trans woman'

Fair do's, I'd say. It would be wonderful, though, if we knew more about the health risks and benefits of long-term oestrogen use for trans women.

Though each human's experience is as unique as pebbles on a beach, anecdotally it seems that the refining process of menopause can bring non-binary and trans people closer to who they really are. In my connection with Samantha, I observed how during their menopause process they've become more spacious in how they can explore their gender and sexual expression:

ATTENDING COMPASSIONATELY TO
THE MENOPAUSE RELATED PAIN IN
MY BODY HAS ACTUALLY HELPED
ME TO FIND OUT MORE ABOUT MY
GENDER, IT BRINGS ME INTO MY
BODY SO I CAN'T IGNORE IT. AS I'M
AGEING I'M REALISING THE WISDOM
OF SEEING THE WHOLE PICTURE – THE
SPHERE INSTEAD OF JUST A CIRCLE.
LEARNING HOW MY MASCULINE AND
FEMININE ASPECTS OPERATE WITHIN
ME HAS BEEN INCREDIBLY HEALING.

All humans are affected by the rhythmical cycles of the moon and the annual seasons, which offer us a simple yet profound guide to life on our journey home. I can't put it better than G. McGregor does:

We all go through changes as humans, it's in the word – transition. We all go through our own unique journeys, emotionally, hormonally, physically, spiritually. We all need to let go of our previous selves in order to boldly step into our authentic selves. Many of us wish that all who identify as men and non-binary folks could discuss these journeys more. Without judgement, without fear and be included in the discussions as having their own unique hormonal, emotional journeys.

This is my own, unique, and valid hormonal journey.

14 Learning to rest

We live in a culture that glorifies productivity above all else. Gross national product must rise year by year, children must achieve ever higher grades, and we must power on through illness. Capitalism built on ever increasing profit, assisted by our old friend patriarchy, means that we can never be still, never be 'enough'. As a species we've lost our rhythm and in the process, we're trashing our beautiful earth, raising anxious children, and have become disconnected from our bodies. Clearly this is not sustainable.

'IT'S EASY IN THEORY TO MAKE EXTRA TIME. BUT THERE HAVE DEFINITELY BEEN GUILT ISSUES FOR ME BECAUSE I "SHOULD BE" WORKING OR DOING, INSTEAD OF RESTING.'

Sharon

We have overwritten our internal code that naturally establishes our cycles of rest and activity. This cycle is visible in the seasons of the year, in the daily circadian rhythm, the breath cycle, and in the menstrual cycle. All humans can recognize it within themselves.

Without rest we cannot be satisfied, because there is no opportunity to connect with our body to notice: *Do I even like this? Does it nourish me?* Without learning what sustains us, we have car crash after car crash, chasing after the elusive feeling of internal goodness. We are not able to reflect or emotionally digest our experiences. We run on empty, endless activity, fuelled by our drug of choice to numb and push through, depleting the body's systems as much as the soul's.

This creates symptoms such as:

- sleep issues
- digestive difficulties
- menopause problems
- period pain
- any condition affected by stress i.e. most illnesses

We are SO tired. Unbelievably tired, because we are endlessly working for an elusive state of satisfaction. Mobile phones and social media won't fix it, but if we were to re-establish our internal rhythm and *trust it*, we might stand a chance.

'AT CERTAIN TIMES, WHEN I WAS STILL WITH MY PARTNER, I WOULD SNEAK AWAY TO WALK IN NATURE AND REST ON PARK BENCHES. IT WAS THE SOLITUDE I CRAVED. SINCE LEAVING MY RELATIONSHIP I HAVE VALUED THE SPACE AND ALONE TIME, AND NOT HAVING TO FEEL THE NEED TO JUSTIFY TIME OUT.'

Sarah

We all *know* we should rest more, but we all feel we can't possibly manage it. We've ingested the message about working harder so deeply from our families, that it can be very difficult to shift. The next time you meet a friend on the street and they ask, 'How're you doing, busy?' see what response you get when you assert, 'I've been lazing around on the sofa, eating chocolate.' Track your own response too. If you're anything like me, you'll notice the impulse to:

- apologize
- justify
- explain how busy I was the day before
- all of the above

As I delved into understanding more about my fatigue in menopause, I found that Chinese medicine ascribes it to kidney yin deficiency. The harder we drive ourselves and use up our resources in our lives, the less energy we have left to manage the transition into menopause. Acupuncturist Juliet Cox tells me:

'Pretty much every woman I see in menopause is kidney yin deficient, but it takes years to manifest through overwork and prolonged stress. It becomes apparent in night sweats, insomnia, increased dryness of skin, dry genitals and extreme tiredness.'

Sound familiar? Chinese medical theory already had Separation figured out 4,500 years ago, pointing to our menopause symptoms as being a result of putting too much energy outwards and not looking after ourselves kindly.

Here are some ways to nourish yourself:

- Commit to periods of daily rest.
- If you have a menstrual cycle, track your Inner Seasons and use your Winter as a time of rest.

- If you don't have a cycle, track with the moon and use the dark moon as your Wintery rest.
- Go slower. Literally move more slowly as you walk about and do tasks.
- Create spaces of quiet in your life.
- Use gentle candlelight in the evenings.
- Reflect on your capacity to receive.

I can recommend getting some validation and encouragement if you decide to rest more; the support of a friend can really help to change the tide of over-activity.

Rest may not mean sleeping. For some people it just doesn't work to sleep in the day, so perhaps we can define deep rest as something that soothes your mind and significantly fills your tanks. It will probably be slow and look like nothing much is happening: yoga nidra (see chapter 15), walking, pottering, gardening, meditating, gentle yoga stretches or painting perhaps. Repetitive movements reduce cortisol, which is why midwives used to knit in the birthing room. It might be a small ritual, like making a proper pot of tea and taking your time to drink it.

Whatever it is, you'll require a little structure to hold yourself to it. Try bolting it on to another existing activity, such as doing some stretches before you get dressed, or block out the time in your diary to make it happen. For eighteen months, I had 'do nothing at all' blocked in my diary every day between 2.30pm and 3pm.

Some of us like to nap, but how long is it before napping interferes with your sleep? A 26-minute nap improved performance in pilots by 34 per cent and alertness by 54 per cent, so perhaps that's the sweet spot for navigating through menopause[1]. It's worth experimenting to see what your own sweet spot is and when to take your nap, so it doesn't mess up your sleep at night.

PRACTICE

Use these prompts as a jumping-off point for journaling or discussion:

- What did you learn you about rest as a child?
- How does this manifest in your capacity to take care of yourself today?
- Is it OK for you to do nothing?
- Commit to a daily period of rest. Starting small is just fine, even 5 minutes.
- Use a lunar chart (see chapter 51) to track the efficacy of your rest whether you nap or rest in some other way, how long for and when.
- See how your mood and energy levels change with different approaches.

Take your foot off the gas.

15 Yoga nidra – the ultimate rest

I first encountered yoga nidra in my weekly yoga class in Watford, but it wasn't until I was in my Separation phase that it became a regular part of my life. I remember walking into the room and being warmly greeted, with the invitation to lie down and get comfy. Tears sprang to my eyes with the relief of being asked to do nothing. Uma started her nidras with:

'You have arrived, there is nothing to do and nowhere to go.'

What bliss for anyone in menopause to hear these words and let them sink in.

I've used yoga nidra almost daily since I found myself in perimenopause, and like many of my clients, it's become the backbone of my menopause self-care. Menopause asks us to slow down, rest and turn our attention inwards; and yoga nidra delivers this plus all the benefits of a meditation practice in an accessible way: no special skills or experience are required, just a quiet place to rest.

There's plenty of research to show how helpful meditation is for anxiety, depression, and pain management.[1] The awareness of our thoughts and body sensation is the gateway to mental and physical wellbeing. So, you'd think we'd all be sitting in meditation for 40 minutes twice a day, but in real life very few of us have a regular meditation practice despite understanding the benefit it brings. If you'd like to meditate but just don't seem to manage it, then you will love yoga nidra. It's a gentle meditation technique that helps us to change gear from 90mph stress-head to a gentle paced, aware relaxation, which rebalances your nervous system and your hormones.

'IN MY MENOPAUSE, NIDRA HAS
BEEN THE DOOR TO DEEP REST AND
GENUINE HEALING.'

Vicki

Yoga means 'union' or 'integration' and nidra means 'sleep'. It can take you from the Beta state of consciousness, which is the ordinary everyday way of being, to Theta, which is the frequency of practised meditators[2]. This is the realm of your subconscious when you're just drifting off to sleep. And sometimes it can even take you to Delta, which is the gateway to the universal consciousness. Without effort.

In classic meditation you anchor your attention on the breath, then often get totally distracted by the stuff in your head. Yoga nidra offers a series of invitations to move your attention around your body, which offers imagery that speaks directly to your unconscious.

'THE NIDRAS ARE JUST LIKE A WARM
COSY PLACE I CAN GO. I LITERALLY
CAN'T FIND THAT ANYWHERE
ELSE. I USED TO FEEL THAT WHEN I WAS
YOUNGER PRIOR TO THE HORMONAL
UPHEAVAL. NIDRAS ARE SUCH A RESPITE
WHEN NOTHING ELSE IS.'

Kathleen

Yoga nidra helps us to integrate, making it easier to activate our creativity, our intuition, and our inner wellness, where we know we are perfect and complete just as we are. Twenty minutes of yoga nidra meditation and maybe you'll be closer to who you aspire to be *as well as* rested and relaxed.

Yoga nidra delivers a beautiful paradox: we are both asleep and awake and we dance along this liminal borderland. It only requires that you let it do its work on you – it is impossible to do it wrong. It's an adaptive practice so that when you need to sleep, you get to sleep, when you need to be awake, you will be awake. And both are OK as your unconscious will still be open to the healing[3].

'THE YEAR BEFORE MENO-
PAUSE I WAS FEELING SCATTERED,
IRRITABLE, WITH POOR MEMORY
AND HORRIBLE FATIGUE. I FEEL
THAT YOGA NIDRA IS THAT FRIEND
THAT YOU CAN ALWAYS LEAN ON
WHEN THE GOING GETS TOUGH
AND WILL ALWAYS SUPPORT YOU NO
MATTER THE CIRCUMSTANCES.'

Bethany

So why isn't everyone doing it? I have a hunch our cultural aversion to doing nothing keeps it as a 'less impressive' sister to meditation because it requires no effort, and we love to measure our success by the amount of effort we put into things and the mastery we achieve. Meditation feels hard where yoga nidra feels easy, and as it's simple and available to everyone right now, it's somehow undervalued.

I have created a yoga nidra for each phase of menopause and for Second Spring, you can read them to yourself or the audio is available for you to download at my website (see Resources, page 392). You can listen to whichever one appeals to you, to evoke the energy of each phase.

- Yoga Nidra for Separation: see page 122
- Yoda Nidra for Surrender: see page 226
- Yoga Nidra for Emergence: see page 317
- Yoga Nidra for Second Spring: see page 356

In each nidra you're going to get comfy, then explore the Seasons in the breath, check in with an inner smile; take a journey of feeling softness all around the body; explore pulsations of this softness; experience the inner journey of Separation, Surrender, Emergence or Second Spring; check back in with an inner smile, the breath and then make your way back into the everyday world. All the time you'll be safe in your resting place.

PRACTICE
- Explore the Yoga Nidra for Separation described in chapter 17.

There is nothing I have to do, there's nowhere to go, I have arrived.

16 The Menstruality Medicine Circle

Menstruality Medicine Circles can give you a sense of how the Seasons have operated in your life, help you to find self-care to suit your needs and giving you a taste of Second Spring. They create a window into the underlying formation of your menopause process to give you a real sense of trust and help you find healing for the challenges you face. The word 'menstruality' refers to the life process from our first period through to menopause;[1] the 'medicine' we receive is our subconscious speaking clearly.

The Menstruality Medicine Circles, created by menstrual educators Red School and further developed at Woman Kind, are a special guided visualization to use whenever you have a question about a symptom or issue, anytime you feel stuck or miserable, or if you feel overwhelmed. They allow access to your deeper wisdom, even if you feel this isn't usually accessible to you. Engaging with a Circle is soothing for the nervous system and for the soul because it gives us orientation, the sense of, 'Oh yes, this is my path!'

'EXPERIENCING THE CIRCLE
HAS BEEN LIFE-CHANGING AND
PROFOUNDLY HEALING. IT HAS
ALLOWED ME TO CONNECT TO
MY WOMB'S WISDOM, DEEPENING
UNDERSTANDING OF MY TRUTH AND
CONNECTION TO THE FEMININE
WITH POTENT, ETHEREAL AND
VISCERAL INSIGHTS THAT OFTEN
TAKE ME BY SURPRISE.'

Chloe

The Circles have been integral to my gathering all the juice possible out of my own menopause process. Without them, I would have struggled to surrender and trust the process. Whenever I get stuck or am in physical or emotional pain, or I want to understand more about what the hell's going on, I use a Circle process to gently guide me into what needs to happen.

'AFTER A CIRCLE I'M MUCH MORE RELAXED AND AT PEACE ABOUT BEING IN PERIMENOPAUSE. I REMEMBER HOW DISTRESSED I WAS WHEN I HAD MY FIRST SYMPTOM — A *22-DAY* CYCLE — BUT THIS MONTH I OVULATED ON DAY *30* AND I'M REALLY AT EASE ABOUT IT. I'M FLOWING MORE WITH THE UNPREDICTABLE NATURE OF MY CYCLE AND NO LONGER CLINGING TO WHAT WAS.'

Cat

What happens in a Circle?

A Circle will give you access into the Life Seasons in a way that is deeply reassuring, bringing deeper understanding of the underlying dynamics and indications for your next steps. There is no wrong way to do it!

To start, you simply formulate a question or intention. It helps if it's as clear as possible, for example:

- Where am I in the menopause process?
- I want to move through this grief.
- I want to learn to love ageing.
- How can I access my strength when I feel so tired?
- Should I take HRT?

Or if there's nothing specific, a question like 'What do I need to take care of here?' can be very powerful.

When you have your question, you settle into the present moment by stepping into the centre of a Circle that you visualize in your mind's eye. The centre is a safe place that you can return to at any time in the process to get an overview of what's happening.

Once there, you'll have a look around at all the Seasons before stepping into Spring, the time of your menarche, through Life Summer, the Autumn of your perimenopause with the phase of Separation, the Winter of your menopause process with Surrender and Emergence, and into your Second Spring. (You might like to refresh your memory of the phases of menopause by revisiting chapter 1.)

For the Circle to be most useful for you, it helps if you can stay present to the thoughts, feelings, sensations and memories as they arise in you and stay curious about what is happening, rather than judging.

Everyone does it differently. You might have access to visualizing things, feeling emotion, sensation in your body, thoughts or memories. This is all information about each Season. Using movement in your Circle is a powerful way to find your medicine; when your body is fluid you just can't stay the same inside. In a relaxed, receptive state, you'll find that while you may touch on your lived experience, the real juice is in your here-and-now experience of the process.

Feeling lost or numb is a very common experience of menopause, which often shows up in a Circle, and it can be helpful to use this as information about your process. Don't feel that you've got anything wrong. Just try to witness your thoughts and feelings without judgement. Whatever arises in your Circle can be used as medicine, even interruptions. For example, if someone disturbs you while you are in the Life Summer of this practice, afterwards you might reflect on how that part of your life was interrupted in everyday life. Getting distracted and thinking about something else while you're in your Circle is also medicine: you can reflect on whether you went unconscious at that time in your life or what's present for you in this Season that you'd rather avoid.

If at any time you find that this process is too overwhelming for you, just back off a little and come back into your body, feeling your feet on the floor and the support around you. You can also return to the centre of the Circle to get some perspective, or step out of it altogether. The purpose is to understand more about what guides you, and you can't do this if you are in a fight, flight or freeze state.

You'll experience each Circle as different, depending on the intention you use, and they can be very surprising. People can experience great variation in the landscape they travel through – all kinds of natural terrain, cityscapes, emptiness, and wild shores, real or imagined.

After your Circle, you will ground your experience by committing to a doable practice that you can manage in your day-to-day life; a little extra kindness to help manifest the medicine. Grounding your Circle with a commitment in your everyday life creates a bridge from the dreamy world of your subconscious into your life. It could be an object or image that you can put by your bed to remind you of the medicine you find, or a commitment to be out in nature every day, or to enjoy a regular date with yourself.

The process of journeying the Circle also has an energetic effect of balancing and healing the cycle all by itself: the experience ripples out energetically, so your life effortlessly changes around you.

The Circle

The Circle is a powerful tool for understanding. However, it is not a substitute for professional therapy. If you are feeling wobbly or experiencing a lot of stress, please get good support and come back to the Circle when things are less charged for you. If you feel very vulnerable during your bleed, then wait until later in your cycle too. If you would prefer to work with somebody, you find details of Circle facilitators in the Resources section (see page 398).

GETTING READY

- Have a journal and pen to hand.
- Make sure you won't be disturbed for 40 minutes.
- Have your intention or question for your Circle prepared, written down if that works for you.
- Turn off your phone ringer and notifications.
- Prepare a little snack and some water for afterwards.

Here's what we're going to do:

1. Get comfy and settle into your body.
2. Check in with your intention or question for the Circle.
3. Once you've settled in, I'll invite you to see the cycle before you and, holding your intention, to step into the centre of the cycle. If you wish, you can close your eyes.
4. You'll land safely in the centre and feel into the landscape around and beyond you.
5. From the centre, you'll step into the Season of Life Spring, from the time of your first period and move through those years, journeying into the Life Summer of your twenties and thirties, into your Life Autumn of perimenopause and Separation, into Life Winter, where you'll move through the menopause phases of Surrender and Emergence, and then into Second Spring of postmenopause. You can spend a minute or two in each Season and phase.
6. Then you'll return to the centre to survey the landscape again.
7. Then finally you will step out of the Circle.
8. You'll come back into the here and now and ground your experience by pondering on some prompts and writing some notes if it suits you.

Once you've got yourself comfy, let's begin.

Taking a deeper breath now, sigh out your out-breath. Do this twice more and notice how your whole body releases as you sigh. Sinking into the earth. Notice how your body is supported, how your back and bum rest on your chair or support. Imagine that deep below the cushions and floor, the warm embrace of the earth is keeping you safe here today.

Bring your intention or question to mind. Say it out loud if you like. Imagine that you could breathe it in like the steam from a bowl of nourishing soup or your favourite tea. Absorb your intention into your system. And holding this awareness, imagine that as you look down at your toes, you could see the beginnings of a different country in front of you. The country of your Life Seasons.

INTO THE CENTRE

Take a big, bold step right into the centre of the cycle, landing safe and secure there with your question. This is a place of safety and wisdom. You can do whatever you need to land safely: visualize yourself dropping an anchor, or imagine safe objects around you perhaps. Know that whenever you need to, if it feels too much, you can return to this centre.

In your own time, imagine you could send your awareness out to survey the Seasons around you. What do you notice? Perhaps you see images, or feel the different qualities of the seasons. Maybe they are indistinct and it's hard to tell them apart. There's no right or wrong way.

Turning about, in your imagination, notice where you feel the Season of Spring, of your teen years from your first period onwards. Orientating yourself towards your Life Spring, and connecting with your intention or question, take a big, bold step into the Season of Spring, landing safely and securely into the time of your first period.

SPRING

As you arrive in your Life Spring, take a breath as you land here, feeling your feet on the ground. Notice how you feel, your emotions and thoughts. What a tender time, full of exploration and discovery as you find out about life and about yourself.

Notice the atmosphere of Spring. There may be body sensation, images, memory – or you may feel nothing at all. Whatever you are aware of, or not, you are doing just fine here. Let yourself be interested in what happens and use your curiosity to observe how it is for you to experience this Life Spring. Maybe there's a colour. You might be alone or you may have other beings around you. Are you feeling a particular emotion?

If you are experiencing something uncomfortable, you could focus on the detail; for example, where its edges are. If it's too much, you can remove yourself to safety and observe the Spring unfold from a little distance, or step into the centre of the cycle to observe. Be super kind to yourself here in this tender Spring and imagine what kind of support you'd love to have here.

Take a moment to feel into a word that captures the quality of your Life Spring: you may like to say it aloud or write it down, staying within the quietness of the Circle.

Then coming back to your Spring landscape, see if there is anything you'd like to do here before we enter Summer. Is there anything you'd like to leave behind? Or perhaps a gift you'd like to receive?

Now you find yourself at the crossover from the Life Spring of your teenage years and the Life Summer. Just notice how it is for you to be here poised on this crossover, and recall your intention or question before stepping into the Summer.

SUMMER

Take some time to land here in your Life Summer – it's the Season of manifesting projects of activity, and of being 'out there' in the world. Get a feel for the bigger energy of this Season. Notice where your attention goes now. If you find yourself distracted, that's OK, come back to your feeling of what this Summer is like and how it impacts you. You may feel more expansive here, excited or overwhelmed.

There may be a body sensation, images, a memory or numbness. Whatever you are aware of, or not, you are doing great. Perhaps you are full of sensation in your body as you experience the move towards creating things in the outside world. Let yourself be interested in the feeling of Summer and stay curious. You might feel an impulse to move or even dance; if so, see where it takes you. Check in with your emotions too.

If you are experiencing something challenging, see if you can stay with it and focus on the detail of the sensation in your body – where it is, perhaps tightness, numbness or tingling. You can always step back into the centre of the cycle to observe and take a few breaths if it feels too much; that's fine too.

What sort of support would you love to have here, in this Summer?

Take a moment to feel into a word that captures the quality of your Life Summer: you may like to say it aloud or write it down.

Coming back to your Summer landscape, see if there is anything you need to do here before we enter Autumn. Is there anything you'd like to leave behind, to let go of? And perhaps there's something you'd like to take with you? You now find yourself at the crossover from Life Summer to Life Autumn of your perimenopause. This can be a powerful moment, and it's important to give yourself space to really notice what this is like for you.

Bring to mind your intention or question you brought to your Circle and take a step into your Life Autumn.

AUTUMN – AND SEPARATION

Take some time to land here in your Life Autumn. Get a feel for the different atmosphere of this Season. It's a Season of decluttering your life. Notice any thoughts, physical or energy sensations, or feelings, and how this Autumnal landscape appears around you. If you are distracted, just take note of it. This is information too. Remember the question that you brought to the Circle and repeat it to yourself. Let yourself be curious about your experience. You're doing beautifully.

Now as you journey through your Life Autumn, you'll feel at some point that you have arrived in the phase of Separation – your perimenopause. You might notice a desire to withdraw, perhaps to curl into yourself somehow, or just a subtle shift in the quality of the environment around you. If you can, be interested if you experience discomfort and notice its quality; is it smooth or spiky? Buzzing or lumpy? Does it have a colour, perhaps? Take a breath. Be soft and kind with yourself here and let yourself have the support you crave. What would that be?

Take a moment to feel into a word that captures the quality of Separation: you may like to say it aloud or write it in your journal.

Coming back to your Autumn landscape, see if there is anything you need to do here before we enter Winter and the phase of Surrender. Is there anything you'd like to leave behind? It could be a belief, or a habit, an attachment to something, or maybe a relation-ship. Is there a gift you'd love to receive? To take with you?

You now find yourself at the crossover from Autumn and Separation into Winter, where you'll encounter Surrender. Just notice how it is for you to be here poised on this crossover.

Now recalling again the question you brought to the Circle and really breathing it in, take a bold step into the Season of Life Winter and Surrender.

WINTER – AND SURRENDER

Take a deep breath in and out as you settle into the phase of Surrender – the place of deep rest and acceptance in this Life Winter. You are now in the depths of your menopause process and finding healing. Notice the differences between Separation and Surrender. Has your body responded? What are your thoughts here? Just notice.

Do you visualize a Wintery landscape around you? What do you need to nourish and soothe yourself? Maybe some colours or an absence of colour show themselves? Let in the softness of Surrender, the peace and quiet. Let yourself receive whatever it is you need to heal, as you fill your spirit. If there is nothing, don't worry, you're doing fine. Doing nothing is excellent medicine especially when you feel lost.

Take a moment to feel into a word that captures the quality of Surrender: you may like to say it aloud, or if you prefer, write it down, staying in the quietness of the Circle.

WINTER – AND EMERGENCE

Moving into Emergence, notice how the new shoots of rising energy make themselves felt. You might feel tingling, want to move again, or your senses may become more alive. Staying curious, notice if you want to move fast, or slow. Do you want to contain this new energy or are you wanting to get busy?

Emergence is a time that asks us to pace ourselves; we're not quite ready to dash out into the world just yet. How could you hold on to your energy and keep it for yourself? You could hug yourself, or breathe into your belly more deeply as you feel your energy build within you?

Take a moment to feel into a word that captures the quality of Emergence: you may like to say it aloud or write it down.

Coming back to the Emergence phase, see if there is anything you need to do here before we enter Second Spring. Is there anything you'd like to leave behind here? It might be a belief, or a habit, an attachment to something, or maybe a relationship. Is there a gift you'd like to give yourself? To take with you into your Second Spring?

You now find yourself at the crossover from the Winter of your menopause and Second Spring completing the cycle you started in your first Spring. What do you notice in yourself at this auspicious time? Is there excitement or dread? A longing to move or perhaps stay quiet and still? You're crossing into a new cycle! Recalling the question you brought to the Circle and really breathing it in, take a bold step into your new cycle and Second Spring.

SECOND SPRING

Take a deep breath in and out as you land here in your Second Spring, on new ground. Get a feel for the different quality of this Season. The clarity of it. The freshness, maybe lightness. How is it different to your first, teenage, Spring? What are you aware of, now, in this different phase of life? Is there body sensation, images, a different emotion?

There might be an energy shift, a smell, or you might hear something. Let yourself move if that feels good, following any impulses from within.

Take a moment to feel into a word that captures the quality of Second Spring: you may like to say it aloud or write it down.

Coming back to Second Spring, look back to where you are in your lived menopause life and give yourself a word of encouragement or love, before you take a bold step back into the centre of the your cycle.

CENTRE

Landing back solidly in the centre once more, take a look around at the journey you have made today. What a journey!

In your imagination, notice any differences in the landscape from when we started. Now it's time to complete your cycle experience, so take a big, bold step right out of the cycle, and back into the here and now. Feeling the floor and chair or the surfaces around you, notice again how they support you and, taking a big breath, sigh to release your out-breath. Do this twice more as you come back into the room.

Now make a gesture or say a word to show to yourself that this Circle experience is complete. Take your time and make any kind of delicious movement that feels good.

Now is a good time to have something to eat and drink, before you reflect on the following questions.

GROUNDING YOUR EXPERIENCE

Once you have completed your Circle process, take some time to ponder and write the answers to the following questions.

- What are the headlines from your Circle?
- What was new information?
- What was charged for you?
- What resources did you encounter that supported you?
- How can you weave a little dose of this medicine into your everyday life?

You can find a link to the audio of The Circle on p. 392.

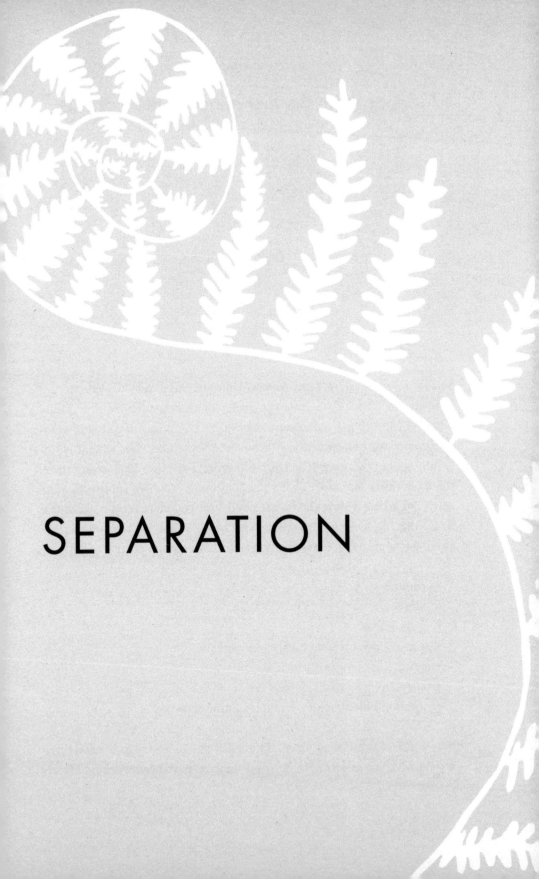

SEPARATION

17 Separation: the first phase of menopause

'IT WAS LIKE WALKING A TIGHT
ROPE OVER A LARGE PRECIPICE.'

Liza

Separation is the call to 'Marie Kondo' your life, except that life decluttering is much, much trickier than reorganizing your knicker drawer. Separation, which equates to perimenopause, marks the beginning of the shift from Summer to Autumn; you know those early September days when the sun is shining, but there's a little chill in the air? The roses are looking tired, the trees dusty and sad? That's the beginning. You feel subtly off, your spirit is looking a little dusty and tired, and you start creating distance from your life, feeling removed or detached. Because it's not comfortable at all, we tend to react negatively as the challenges appear:

- tiredness
- stress
- feeling lost
- you see what is not working in your life
- grief
- anger
- random illness, injury, and misfortune show up

You will feel tired. Very tired. This does not mean there is something wrong with you necessarily, it means that you have been working bloody hard at being alive. My punt is that if the world supported menstrual cycle awareness and we could easily follow our natural need to rest for a few days every month, we would not be so knackered at menopause. Unfortunately, many of us arrive at the gateway on our knees already, under-resourced to face the challenges that await us.

The hormonal changes at menopause make us super sensitive to stress. It's so unfair! We also become highly sensitized to noise, foods, and all kinds of things, just at the point where we are experiencing seismic physical and psychological change. Added to this, high stress levels will make every single menopause symptom worse. It's totally unfair!

Separation also makes us feel lost and confused. This has a psychological purpose, because we have to lose ourselves in order to find a juicier version of ourselves in Second Spring. It can feel very frightening for sure, and it can be a comfort to know that you are held in a process here. It's very uncomfortable because as humans, we like to know where we're going, to be in control, including a satnav to guide us and a nice Instagram photo of our beautiful destination.

Think of it as the archetypal hero's journey, where the narrative takes us away from our safe home and sends us into the wilds of nature, where we are required to use our courage and intuition to get the help we need, so we can return home changed. There are many, many stories you can use as a guide; for example, Hansel and Gretel left their family and got lost in the woods, gathering their wisdom before they could follow the trail of breadcrumbs back home. Red Riding Hood faced the wolf. In the Russian Baba Yaga story, Vasilisa had her doll to help her complete the tasks before she went home to set fire to her family . . . There's a story for everyone! All of them say the same thing: 'You will be lost, but you will return wiser, stronger and happier.'

One of the gifts of Autumn is discernment. You are treated to a clear view of what is not working in your life. This often brings divorce, crisis, and rage. This is part of the de-cluttering process that is necessary. Mostly it hurts.

'AT 45, I CONCLUDED THAT I COULD NOT STAY WITH THE MAN I WAS MARRIED TO BECAUSE I COULDN'T BE MYSELF. I HAD FOUR CHILDREN TO SUPPORT, SO I WORKED OUT A PLAN OF HOW I COULD PAY ALL THE BILLS AND SUPPORT THE CHILDREN IF HE WOULDN'T SUPPORT US. I WAS 48 WHEN I TOLD HIM OUR MARRIAGE WAS OVER. HE WAS ABUSIVE IN MANY WAYS, SO IT WAS QUITE A SHIFT FOR ME TO ACTUALLY SAY I'VE HAD ENOUGH. IT TOOK ANOTHER EIGHTEEN MONTHS BEFORE HE ACTUALLY LEFT THE HOUSE, AND THAT WAS THE START OF MY EMPOWERMENT. THEN WHEN I WAS 50, I FOUND YOGA. WHETHER IT WAS THE YOGA OR ME BEING POSTMENOPAUSAL, I STARTED MAKING DIFFERENT DECISIONS, AND I CAME INTO MY POWER.'

Cryn

Historically, menopausal women have been ridiculed as either mad or angry, but as we'll be dealing with the former possibility in more detail in chapter 20, let's deal with the anger now. I'd like to reassess that judgement from a feminist angle and suggest that there are many things in our lives that we are entirely justified in being bloody furious about. The endless sexism, the way we have messed up our planet and the fallout from that, the opportunities lost, the abuse and trauma, financial loss. Maybe we should be even angrier? Anger is the precursor for change, for movement, and without it, we are in stasis. Imagine if our anger were continually stuffed down and not expressed? It doesn't bear thinking about the pain that this causes in terms of depression and as repressed anger is also a contributor to heart disease, stroke, anxiety, and can even shorten your life.

I find myself particularly enraged by the way menopause is ridiculed by people of all genders. It denies us the right to our fear, our rage. It cheats us from the reality of this extraordinary shift in consciousness. Not that I want to eliminate humour, far from it – there's a daftness that arises to pierce pomposity and call out the bullshit. I long for a time when Separation is dignified as an important rite of passage, and we'll be given the peace we need to pay attention to this magnificent transformation.

It's a bit like when you're going on holiday. Before leaving, all the long-avoided admin and domestic tasks acquire a sudden urgency. In menopause, time and again, women share that they have had accidents, injuries, family crisis, financial crisis, and all kinds of random stuff that makes us say, 'This can't be related to menopause, can it?' What's happening is that old wounds are demanding our attention before we move on. Call it emotional admin: issues around vulnerability, early attachment issues, security, abuse, and trauma all surface in various guises for us to have another go at healing a bit more. This is exhausting to say the least, but it's essential to remember it's not a punishment. I am saddened when I hear people say, 'I think it's hurting because I'm not doing it right!' Transforming into something else is a *tender* process, and it's supposed to be messy.

As menopause is a natural time of decluttering, the flip-side of this is grief. Grief for the things that are passed, things you have not done, things that you have done and would rather you hadn't. Youth has gone. There's no getting around this and inevitably you will feel a degree of sadness about it. Grief and sadness are just part of the process and if you can honour them, you'll feel so much lighter on the other side.

In the graphic of the Life Seasons on page 29, you'll have seen that the phases look like nice orderly slices of cake for you to munch your way through. In real life, growth doesn't happen neatly. You'll find yourself in Separation one moment and Surrender the next, with whiffs of Emergence arriving in the morning and a side of Second Spring with your dinner. When you look back in retrospect from your Second Spring clarity, you'll probably be able to track how the broad arc of the phases played out over the years, but meanwhile, day to day, they will *all* be present in your daily life.

The fabulous power of the phases is that once you can recognize and name them to yourself, you can bypass any self-criticism and go straight to the self-care they demand. I remember one night when I was desperately trying to marshal my children to the dinner table to eat the food I had resentfully made and didn't want to eat; I realized I was about to lose it and, for once, caught myself: 'Aha! Hello Separation!' Knowing that the medicine for Separation is to have space to myself to withdraw, I disappeared and left them to it. A small domestic incident for sure, but isn't that what life is made up of – a series of small incidents?

Separation is the longest phase of menopause and arguably the hardest. The following chapters in this section are devoted to aspects that you may encounter, along with practical self-help and enquiry to deepen your relationship with yourself, and move through it all with style.

PRACTICE

- Use the Circle (see chapter 16) with an intention that addresses your current symptoms.
- Rest with the Yoga Nidra for Separation, which you'll find next.

If it's messy, you're doing it right.

Yoga Nidra for Separation

This nidra will give you about 15 minutes of deep rest. Find a cosy space where you can recline undisturbed, with all the cushions and blankets you need, and as you read the practice through to yourself, let yourself be open to what feels good for you. You might like to prop the book on a cushion, for example, so your arms and hands can relax ...

GETTING READY

Welcome to the practice of yoga nidra.

Welcome to this safe, protected place of rest, your true home.

Just arriving here is enough, we've burned the to-do list and the hard part is over.

There is no wrong way to do this.

This is all just an invitation – if there's anything that doesn't sit well with you, you can let it go.

GETTING COMFY

The intention of this practice is to accept the process of Separation.

Hang up your 'do not disturb' sign, turn off your phone, and create a space to rest, gathering all the cushions and blankets you need to recline comfortably.

Wriggle around to find a position where your shoulders can release a bit more, softly settling back ...

Releasing the jaw with a yawn or a sigh.

Sinking into your resting place.

Letting your eyes soften.

Noticing the sounds beyond the place you are resting in.

Noticing the sounds in the space around you.

Drawing your attention closer to notice the sound of your breath.

THE SEASONS IN THE BREATH

Noticing the breath, the uniqueness of each breath, just soft and effortless.

How each breath holds the Seasonal cycle, each one different and yet the same.

The start of the in-breath is the dawn of Spring,

Coming into the fullness of Summer,

Then releasing into the Autumn of the out-breath,

And the quiet of Winter at the end of the out-breath.

Notice how the Seasons roll effortlessly through the breath, the inevitability of it,

The way your belly rises with the in-breath,

Always followed by the release and emptying of the out-breath;

Spring and Summer bringing you out into the world, and Autumn and Winter bringing you home to yourself ...

Name the Seasons of the breath for a few more cycles, with the belly rising and falling.

For a few breaths, notice the turn of the breath, where you easily shift from fullness to release.

INNER SMILE

Take a moment to imagine that something good is coming your way, a pleasing sense of anticipation; good stuff is coming towards you ...
Notice how this feels in your body:
Like an inner smile.

ALLOWING SOFTNESS THROUGH THE BODY

You're going to take a journey, visiting places in the body and imagining they could each in turn soften and release, in their own way.
Softening between the eyebrows ...
Softening and releasing the jaw, the tongue and throat ...
A wash of softness travelling down the right arm from the shoulder to each fingertip,
A wash of softness travelling down the left arm from the shoulder to each fingertip,
Releasing and softening the torso from collar bone, through the heart, the navel and down to the pubic bone;
A wash of softness travelling down the right leg from the hip to the tip of each toe,
A wash of softness travelling down the left leg from the hip to the tip of each toe,
Your bum just lets go ...
Then the base of the spine upwards is washed by a wave of softening and releasing all up the whole of the back,
The neck can let go of the head,
The softness washes over the temples, the eyes, cheeks, nose and jaw,
The whole body softens and releases.

PULSATIONS

And as the breath comes in, notice how the body expands slightly, taking up more space, then as the breath leaves, the body settles more comfortably back into its place.
Breathing in to create space and breathing out to land even more comfortably home.
Follow these pulsations for a few breath cycles.
Now holding the experience of both expansion and coming home safe at the same time, how would that be? To have awareness of both together?
Take a moment to feel this.

INNER JOURNEY OF SEPARATION

Imagine that you could journey down inside, into the pelvic bowl ... Where you find you can rest in a safe, comfortable nest, with just the right kind of softness, just the right cushions and blankets for you to rest perfectly.
Look how the gleaming, resilient structure of the pelvis encircles you and holds you safe, free from worries or cares. You are protected here.

Deep in the centre lies a precious fruit, glowing, ripening, blushing golden in her fullness. And as you rest safely here, this golden fruit shines out a beautiful golden light to fill the pelvic bowl, allowing you to be both separate and safe, separate and safe, a golden light surrounding you all about.

The soft golden light gently burns off what no longer serves you, letting you rest calmly in your Separation. Resting quiet and safe, deep in your pelvic bowl, nourished as you effortlessly release.

THE SEASONS IN THE BREATH

Noticing the breath once more ...
How each breath holds the Seasonal cycle, each cycle different and yet the same:
The start of the in-breath the dawn of Spring,
Coming into the fullness of Summer,
Then releasing into the Autumn of the out-breath,
And the quiet of Winter.
Notice how the Seasons roll effortlessly through you, the inevitability of it,
The way your belly rises with the in-breath,
Always followed by the release and emptying of the out-breath.

INNER SMILE

Take another moment to imagine that something good is coming your way:
A warm openness ready to receive goodness.
Notice how this feels in your body:
Like an inner smile.

RETURNING TO THE HERE AND NOW

Noticing now the sound of your breath,
Expanding your attention to the sounds in the room around you ...
The sounds beyond the room as you come back into the here and now;
Start to expand your awareness of where you are, looking around at your space ...
Start to stretch and move, yawn and wriggle as you come back to the everyday world.

As we close this practice of yoga nidra, accept the process of Separation.

Wide awake, wide awake and present.
Let yourself move gently from this yoga nidra, giving yourself space before you move back into your everyday life.

Congratulations on giving yourself this rest.

You can find a link to the audio for this nidra on p. 392.

18 The gifts of Separation

Despite Separation being gruelling, there is hard-won gold to be found from bringing kindness to the physical and emotional challenges. If you are open to receiving gifts in Separation, you are already doing brilliantly at developing the positive mindset that will help you heal. Here are some of the gifts you might find:

Discernment: it is so clear what's worth the effort and what is not.

Truth: we know the truth and can communicate it clearly (no filters!).

Finding our NO: we can say no to the outside world and yes to ourselves.

Knowing ourselves: we are invited to pay attention and build a relation-ship with our true needs and our inner life, which reasserts itself here.

Intuition: our inner voices speak loud in dreams and sudden knowing.

Meeting our negativity: we meet our inner critic (see chapter 33) who has some interesting info for us – albeit delivered in a shouty way.

Strength: we get to build the muscle of holding tension – grrr! This is not the kind of tension where your shoulders are up around your ears; this is softly holding the conflict between both our inner and outer world, so we can validate our feelings while still operating in the real world at work. See chapter 63, 'Holding the charge', for more on this.

Losing it: we also practise losing the plot, which is an extremely useful skill. No one ever in the whole world made a transition by holding it all together; this is the time to release control and let the winds of change whip up our knickers.

PRACTICE

You might like to explore this question as a journaling prompt, as a discussion with friends, to dream into or as inspiration for a creative project.

- Which of the Separation gifts can you recognize in yourself?
- Rest with the Yoga Nidra for Separation (see pages 122–124).

I am perfectly imperfect just as I am.

19 Is this it?

If you are 45 or older and you're experiencing four or more of the things in the list below, you could be perimenopausal – aka in the Separation phase of menopause. Take this quiz to find out!

1. Are you pissed off? Do those things that irritated you before your period, now irritate you *all* the time?
2. Do you find you can't just 'put up' with things that are wrong for the sake of a quiet life anymore?
3. If your menstrual cycle was regular, does it now vary in length each month?
4. Have your periods become like a blood bath, with you changing pads every hour or more often?

5. Have your periods practically disappeared?
6. Do you get hot at night, but not because you're feeling 'hot'?
7. Do you feel an inexplicable sense of grief and cry over nothing?
8. Do you fantasize about running away from your life to live on your own?
9. Do you feel lost or bewildered?
10. Have you lost your passion for your work and find it hard to care?
11. Do you experience non-specific anxiety that seems to hang around longer than usual?
12. Have you developed tender boobs all of a sudden?
13. Are your jeans weirdly tight, even though you haven't eaten more than usual?
14. If you have them, are your children less fascinating than they used to be?
15. If you haven't had children, are you grieving or fantasizing about babies that might have been?
16. What's it called? Errr, brain fog! Do you forget why you walked into the room?
17. Do you long to nap, all the time?
18. Are your bullshit detectors set to high?
19. Are you finally understanding how to say NO to the things you don't want in your life?

Separation is a time when our physical and emotional vulnerabilities tend to catch up with us as we are more sensitized to everything. We are starting a process of change. Instead of freaking out about these changes, try to regard them as your body asking you to slow down and be gentler with yourself. It's a wake-up call to let you know that it's time to change the way you relate to yourself now that your hormonal picture is changing.

'THE TIREDNESS WAS PUT DOWN TO MENOPAUSE BUT TURNED OUT TO BE HYPOTHYROIDISM. I HAVE MUCH MORE ENERGY NOW I'M ON MEDICATION.'

'Jane'

It is common for pre-existing imbalances to show up in your forties. While a blood test will not tell you if you are perimenopausal when you're over 45, go to your doctor to check out any big changes in your cycle just to rule out other possibilities, and engage professional complementary therapists for advice too if you wish. It's easy for symptoms of other issues to be cloaked and assumed to be perimenopause.

The levels of your follicle-stimulating hormone, or FSH, are the definitive test for menopause. Sometimes doctors are reluctant to give you this test if you're over 45, but if you're concerned it's definitely worth asking about. Here's the low-down:

- If you still have your menstrual cycle, day 3 is the recommended day for blood tests.
- If you don't have a menstrual cycle, it can be any time of the month.
- Hormone levels fluctuate with stress levels, so it's a good idea to get a second test a month later.
- It's important to have your results interpreted by a professional, but as a guide, FSH levels above 10 to 12 mIU/mL may indicate you are approaching perimenopause. While 30 to 40 mIU/mL or above is usually taken to indicate that you are in menopause.
- Some doctors will follow up with a serum estradiol concentration test to measure the amount of estradiol in your blood.

If you can't access an FSH test, you might want to explore DUTCH advanced hormone testing, which will provide an in-depth look at your hormone picture. It's a comprehensive hormone test that will give you a full picture of what's going on and will need to be interpreted by a professional. They can be ordered through a nutritionist or, at the time of writing, directly from dutchtest.com.

The main psychological tone of perimenopause is feeling lost. This feels like shit – but ultimately it sets you free to be present in the moment and have *a lot* of pleasure. Your mission is to develop kindness towards yourself as you find your way. This is a big thing.

PRACTICE
- Take a moment to place your hands on your lower belly and feel your breath as it moves in your torso.
- Ask yourself, what is it that I need right now? How can I be kind here?
- Find a way to give yourself this gift.

My feelings are valid, even when I don't understand why I feel them.

20 It feels like you're going mad, but in fact you're growing sane

One of the most common ways that Separation announces itself is the feeling that you're not quite yourself. Typically, we feel the need to withdraw from things that previously gave us pleasure and meaning. Imagine the kind of efficient office manager, who everyone usually relies on, going into a meltdown at a minor admin hiccup, or a saintly health worker struggling to care about her patients, or a writer (ahem) who finds she can't string a sentence together. These types of crisis announce the beginning of the Life Autumn, in which we start to see the truth more clearly, and identities that no longer serve us start to crack.

'I SERIOUSLY THINK AT TIMES I AM GOING MAD, BUT AT THE SAME TIME THERE IS A GROWING SENSE THAT IT'S THE REST OF THE WORLD THAT'S CRAZY AND I SEEM TO BE GOING SANE.'

Birgitte

Let me explain. Separation is a sensitive time when we naturally want to retreat into ourselves. Our energy is low and hormone fluctuations are playing out in our mood and physical health. This challenges our capacity to do pretty much anything, but especially when we engage with outdated roles – because they are completely *exhausting*. As the role fits us less and less well, it takes more and more energy to sustain it.

It's easy for our jobs to become our identifiers, isn't it? The caring one, the efficient one or the articulate one, especially when we are rewarded for them, because that's easier than holding the complex, contradictory, and cyclical person we are. We learn to hold these roles early in life, and they can become particularly rigid when our parents only allowed us to express a narrow band of behaviour.

Once the menopause transition gets underway and you're moving towards a different, more authentic way of being where you can inhabit more of yourself, the old roles start to feel increasingly uncomfortable. It's as though we're waking up to the discomfort of the tight-fitting role and it's time for it to be shrugged off. As Uma Dinsmore-Tuli, author of *Yoni Shakti*, memorably said: 'It takes your head out of your arse.' We may have learned the necessity of being good and staying small when younger because this keeps us safe, but now it is time to grow. If you've been tootling along for twenty-five years or so in this role, it can feel very frightening, but in order to change you will have to shed your snakeskin. It's a scary prospect. Remember, it's not our core cracking up, it's the more superficial, outdated roles falling away, and this allows us to be 'more' of ourselves. This process of coming back to our core self can also bring sanity; for example, Samantha, one of my interviewees, was able to *stop* taking anti-psychotics at menopause, telling me: 'Menopause saved my life! I feel like I'm becoming who I truly am.'

Interestingly, many women develop a literal, physical itch at this time; perhaps it's the body feeding back to us that it's time to burst out of playing small?

Another way you might feel you're going mad is when Separation announces her arrival with a sudden, inexplicable anxiety bursting from nowhere. One day you're rocking along more or less OK; the next you're plagued with catastrophic thoughts, a racing heart and searing sweats.

'MY WIFE THOUGHT I'D LOST THE PLOT. OVERNIGHT I CHANGED FROM BEING A ROCK IN OUR FAMILY, TO BEING A TEARY, SWEATY HEAP!'

Nadine

Anxiety is an aspect of our stress response and it can be almost impossible to pick apart if it's to do with the hormonal dips or being triggered by old issues, tiredness, the many life-pressures you're dealing with, or fear of becoming that scary monster–'the perimenopausal woman'.

My sense from observing clients is that having been operating at unsustainable levels of plate-spinning for decades, when Separation calls us to slow down, it *is* terrifying. Our minds become filled with 'But I can't stop', 'I have too much to do', and the fear of what will happen when we let go is immense.

Rather than get lost in overthinking, because we may never be absolutely sure of the 'why', it can be helpful to focus on the 'how'. First, you'll need to soothe your nervous system by stepping back a bit so you can think more clearly; maybe use one of the nidra meditations or go out and connect with nature in a way that's pleasing for you. Once the emotional charge is reduced enough for you to feel more stable, have a look at chapter 45, on healing wounds with Tara Brach's the RAIN meditation. This will help you to begin to integrate what you're feeling and soothe yourself even more. Once RAIN or some other suggested practice is helping you manage better, have a look at the table in chapter 3 and make one small change in your diet.

PRACTICE

You might like to explore these questions in your journal, or by talking with friends or in a circle, to dream into or as inspiration for a creative project.

- What did your parents praise you for when you were a child?
- Are you still trying to earn acceptance/feel good enough/worthy enough now by taking on particular roles today?
- Dream into your ideal day by journaling, drawing, daydreaming or chatting with a friend. What would that look, feel, taste, and smell like?
- Imagine your perfect day: can you identify a small aspect of it and commit to bringing it into your life every day? It might just be something like enjoying a mindful cup of tea, laughing at a movie or gazing out at nature?
- Rest with the Yoga Nidra for Separation (see pages 122–124).

I am the sane one.

21 There are some symptoms that no one tells you about

Mention menopause and most people will think of hot flushes[1], the butt of most menopause jokes. Though flushes and sweats are seriously debilitating for some, they are at least well known, unlike the wide range of sensitivities and issues that may show up in the menopause transition.

> 'I HAD NO IDEA THAT ALL THESE SYMPTOMS, WHICH ALL SEEMED TO COME AT ONCE, WERE SYMPTOMS OF PERIMENOPAUSE.'
>
> *Sandra*

Another part of menopause that is not widely understood is the immense *variety* of ways our bodies change. Because the huge range of midlife challenges is not fully understood, it can be a great surprise when someone finds herself suddenly overcome by brain fog at the age of 45, and if it's unexpected then the logical response is panic and fear.

My first inkling of perimenopause showing up was that the soft padding on the soles of my feet and on my hands disappeared. It felt like my bones were grinding into the earth with every step. In a real way, I *have* lost my softness and the cushioning in my earth connection, but I am grounded and connected through my bones more strongly than ever before. I feel part of the earth; her seasons are my seasons. Loss of tissue on the feet is *extremely* common in perimenopausal women, as the reduction in oestrogen levels affects the production of collagen. No wonder plantar fasciitis, which causes pain to the heel and sole of the foot, is rife in perimenopause. If more people knew to expect this, and wore comfy shoes before the pain started, we could prevent a great deal of suffering.

Much stress and anxiety can be avoided if we understand that these weird symptoms are tied up with the transition into menopause and that they can arise from the stress we're carrying at this sensitive time of change. Our bodies demand that we change our ways; we simply cannot carry on as we have been doing, it's just not sustainable.

'IT'S LIKE NOTHING ELSE WHEN IT'S HAPPENING IN YOUR OWN BODY. *EVERYTHING* CHANGES. HORMONAL SHIFTS MESS WITH YOUR PERCEPTION — A FEW DAYS BEFORE MY PERIOD EVERYTHING WOULD SEEM BLEAK AND SAD AND I'D OVERREACT BEFORE, BUT THEN I FELT LIKE THIS ALL THE TIME. I WAS BLEEDING AT IRREGULAR TIMES, AND EVERYTHING BECAME ABSOLUTELY SHOCKING AND DISORIENTATING.'

Kathleen

How about this for a list of surprising symptoms:

tingling extremities

misphonia and tinnitus

urinary tract infections

dizziness

new allergies and sensitivities to food   digestive problems

heart palpitations and panic attacks

bleeding gums   restless legs

loss of tissue to feet, hands and generally around

aching joints   sore breasts

bad breath

joint stiffness   reduced muscle mass

taste sensitivities

burning tongue

breasts growing bigger

weird smelling sweat   stress incontinence

itchy skin

hair loss

Please don't freak out – if you experience any of these, you are not alone. Many can be managed and are caused by stress in the body, there's even some evidence that a higher exposure to trauma will worsen your symptoms[2]. Nearly all of them will improve by managing your stress or just melt away in Second Spring. However, it's always worth getting worrisome symptoms checked out by your doctor; don't assume everything is menopause. Perhaps most important of all, the symptoms that are showing up for you *do not define your identity.* My teenage kids are forgetful, my male partner has weird aches, and many people become hyper-sensitized for a variety of mysterious reasons, not just in menopause. Your body speaking to you in these ways just means that you are human and deserve good care, from yourself most of all.

'I WAS ALWAYS RELIEVED WHEN I COULD PUT A SYMPTOM SUCH AS HOT FLUSHES DOWN TO MENOPAUSE AND THAT WE COULD VIEW IT AS A RISE IN GOOD ENERGY WITH THE BODY TRANSITIONING INTO THE MOST POWERFUL TIME IN YOUR LIFE. THINGS LIKE HEADACHES SURPRISED ME, AS I NEVER EVER HAD ANY, SO THEN THIS WAS A BODY MESSAGE TO SAY HEY IT'S HAPPENING, BE AWARE OF IT, EMBRACE IT, FOLLOW ITS COURSE TO ITS BRIGHT, SHINY, GLITTERING END.'

Sarah

PRACTICE

A great technique to avoid catastrophizing about symptoms is to let them speak to you directly. Grab yourself 20 minutes of uninterrupted time and imagine that the symptom was a person or creature so you can have a chat with them, either out loud or written in your journal.

- Decide which symptom to focus on.
- In your imagination, sit them on the chair or cushion in front of you.

- Give them a name.
- Tell them how you feel about them.
- Listen to how they respond.
- You might like to ask supplementary questions like 'What do you need me to know?',
- 'How can I support you?' or 'How are you trying to help me?'

A symptom does not define who you are, you get to choose who you want to be.

22 What about early menopause?

Around 1 in 100 women in the UK experience menopause symptoms under the age of 40[1], which is known as premature menopause. It can drive you right to your edge if you were planning to have a family later in your reproductive life, bringing misery and significant mental and psychological challenges with it. If you are postnatal with small children, an early menopause can bring you to your knees, and support and advice are often patchy for younger women.

Early menopause goes by the miserable moniker of 'premature ovarian insufficiency', which is certain to trash your self-esteem.[2] Though often no particular cause is found, it can be genetic so it's good to ask your female relatives about what age their menopause showed up. Other causes can be autoimmune diseases, TB or mumps[3]. Unlike women in the usual age range for menopause (45 to 55), if you are in your thirties, having a raised follicle-stimulating hormone level over a couple of blood tests *will* demonstrate early menopause. It's a good idea to have tests for low thyroid too, as the symptoms are remarkably similar: depression, sleep problems, weight gain, brain fog and hot flushes. Don't assume it's early menopause; do get tests to confirm it. The menstrual cycle is a sensitive health barometer and imbalances show up quickly in our cycles, so it may be the sign that something else is awry and needing attention.

'I'M EXPERIENCING AN EARLY NATURAL MENOPAUSE AND WITH A FULL-ON CAREER, PRE-TEENS AND TEENAGERS I'VE NEVER FELT MORE STRETCHED — LOSING MY ENERGY LEVELS AT THIS TIME HAS BEEN DEVASTATING.'

'Rebekah'

In the long term, an early menopause contributes to the risk of osteoporosis and cardiovascular disease, so oestrogen replacement is often advised into your early fifties. The psychological phases of menopause will still be operating whatever age it arrives, but the effect of having low energy and an inward focus is very different at the age of 32 than it would be at 48, creating all sorts of different tensions in your life. Also, sometimes ovulatory cycles wake up and kick back in again for reasons unknown and 8 per cent of women with early menopause will get pregnant.[4] Don't forget that pregnancy is still possible today with egg donation and surrogacy, and there are also experimental attempts to reverse premature menopause. The good news is that there is support available: Earlymenopause.com, for example, has some great resources.

'BEFORE I KNEW I WAS IN EARLY MENOPAUSE, I FELT COMPLETELY UNLIKE MYSELF — LYING ON THE SOFA FOR AN AFTERNOON, MY USUAL ZEST, GET UP AND GO, COMPLETELY GONE. BUT THEN, I HAD BEEN RAISING TWO YOUNG KIDS AND MANAGING THE HOME WHILE WORKING FOR ABOUT 10 YEARS, SO A GOOD REST WAS NEEDED.'

Jessica

PRACTICE

- Talk to your mum and/or female relatives about their menopause experience.
- Find other women who are experiencing the same issues on social media or forums.
- Find ways of expressing your feelings safely.

Choose to love yourself, even when the universe has other plans.

23 What about induced menopause?

Many women arrive at menopause after having an operation. If you've had your womb removed – a hysterectomy – it's fairly common to keep your ovaries, where your progesterone and oestrogen are made; but even so, you still may experience an early menopause, or even a later one, as menopause mentor Bryn Truett-Chavez described to me:

Though they had taken my womb, my ovaries and everything at 30, in my sixties I went through menopause; hot flushes and everything. I took it as this is my soul's journey, the part where you stand in your own truth and say, "I'm claiming my sovereignty; I'm claiming my wise years." At nearly 70, it feels even more exciting.

Without a womb you won't be having periods, so it can be confusing to know whether you are experiencing menopause or what the hell's going on. If you have had your ovaries and fallopian tubes removed as well as your womb, cheerily known as a 'total hysterectomy and bilateral salpingo oophorectomy' or 'TAH and BSO', the effect is immediate and brutal and oestrogen levels are floored within 24-hours[1]. Generally, HRT – both micronized progesterone and bioidentical estradiol – are recommended, starting immediately after your operation[2].

But there is an alternative view where if we understand that menopause is an initiation into something bigger, *and are given time to heal,* there is deep medicine available to us even in surgical menopause. Sarah Miller, founder of Embodiments Dance, Drum, Circle, had a hysterectomy following a cancer diagnosis:

> *I have found that this framing of my menopause as a sacred rite of passage – as an opportunity of huge growth – has meant that what- ever I am experiencing, is okay. At least most of the time. When you understand your menopause as an initiation into the next phase of your life, you have some perspective on what you are experiencing and can see value in the challenges. The current discourse on menopause is often fear-based and controlling and you may feel you are a victim. But reframe this! Reframe yourself as an initiate – one who is becoming a Wise Woman, a Maga, Magissa – the Magician. Own this experience as yours, however it looks. This is a time for stepping into your power.[3]*

Some of the worst symptoms are the ones that affect the way you think, with concentration, mood and memory being particularly affected. Campaigner Diane Danzebrink has written movingly about how the lack of information about surgical menopause, which nearly cost her life when the 'feeling of blackness and sheer hopelessness' descended.[4] She turned down HRT at first because she was put off by it being made of pregnant mares' urine and her doctors didn't inform her about plant-based, bioidentical HRT. Her experience powers her passionate campaign to educate medics and employers about the process of menopause and her petition Make Menopause Matter has reached more than 100,000 signatures at the time of writing.[5] She also has an excellent Facebook community where you can tap into support for surgical menopause.

'I HAD DECIDED TO NOT HAVE IVF IN MY EARLY FORTIES, WHEN I WAS UNABLE TO CONCEIVE, BECAUSE I DID NOT FEEL I WANTED CHILDREN THAT DESPERATELY BUT DID HAVE TO DEAL WITH SOME GRIEF OVER NEVER BEING ABLE TO HAVE THEM. I EMBARKED ON CREATIVE PROJECTS WHICH REALLY HELPED TO BIRTH SOMETHING FROM DEEP WITHIN. TWO YEARS AGO, I HAD A HYSTERECTOMY, DUE TO SUSPECTED WOMB LINING CANCER. BIOLOGICALLY IT MEANT THAT WAS DEFINITELY THAT ON THE CHILD FRONT. I AM GLAD TO SAY THAT I STILL SENSE THE MENSTRUAL CYCLE QUITE STRONGLY AND CHART IT VIA THE MOON.'

'Fanella'

Removing your womb is a big deal; for some it's a blessed relief, for others it's as though their very femininity has been cut out. It's important to remember that you are more than your organs, and, that the energy of the womb is still present in the pelvic bowl, even if the physical womb has gone. The energy of the womb is grounding, generating our creativity and sexuality, and this is *still* available to you. The Womb Journey visualization on pages 147–148 will help you deepen your connection to the energetic qualities available in your pelvic bowl.

There are implications to having a hysterectomy, especially if you feel it has been forced rather than wholeheartedly chosen. The medical profession can often seem rather cavalier about whipping out 'useless' wombs; after all, you don't need this troublesome organ anymore, right? Mandy Chadwick recounted how when her doctor recommended a hysterectomy to resolve her heavy bleeding and abnormal cells following her divorce, she told him:

> *My uterus is my second heart. It radiates female energy and I wish to do all I can to restore its function.'*

Needless to say, Mandy still has her womb today and went on to fully restore her cycle before her menopause began at 58.

Preparing for surgery

Like any loss, the quality of the departure sets the tone for the grieving and recovery. If you are preparing for a hysterectomy, you might want to explore what your womb represents for you and what needs to happen for you to release her with grace. Melanie Rossiter, author of *Reclaiming Feminine Wisdom*, says of her experience:

> *I wanted to release my womb in a way that would release the trauma that it had been through and to clear up the mess.* [6]

In her book, Melanie describes how, before her hysterectomy, she created a beautiful ritual to release her womb in peace and most importantly gave herself time to grieve and process her feelings; this lead to a Wintery inward focus that ultimately helped her to move on to a new way of being. Her suggestions for a ritual include:

- womb meditation
- journaling about your fears
- journaling your gratitude for your womb
- writing your womb a letter
- burying an object that represents your womb and creating a ritual around that
- creating an artwork, painting, song or dance

If you're reading this having had a hysterectomy that you were not prepared for and want to make your peace in retrospect, creating a ritual now is a beautiful way to complete the cycle of grief.

'CELEBRATION WAS ANOTHER VITAL BLESSING OF THIS SURGICAL MENOPAUSE JOURNEY. IN PREPARATION FOR LOSING MY WOMB I INITIATED AND WAS GIFTED WITH WOMB CEREMONIES. THESE WERE PROFOUND OPPORTUNITIES TO BE WITH THE EXPERIENCE OF WOMB LOSS, TO SURRENDER TO THE PROCESS I WAS UNDERGOING, AND TO MAKE SACRED THIS SACRIFICE OF MY WOMB.'

Sarah Miller, founder of Embodiments Dance, Drum, Circle[7]

PRACTICE

- Use the Womb Journey meditation on pages 147–148 to connect to your womb or womb space.
- If you are preparing for or have experienced a hysterectomy, there are three aspects of letting go to be acknowledged: expressing gratitude, releasing, and grieving. All need to be explored and expressed in a way that feels safe and comfortable for you.
- Would you like part or all of this letting-go process to be witnessed? If so, by whom? Friends, a mentoring group, your therapist?
- Would you like someone to hold space for you to do this letting go? If so, see the Therapies section on page 397 for someone to help you with that.
- If you prefer to work through this alone, what medium do you prefer? Writing, painting, crafting, singing, dancing? What's your comfy place?

I reframe myself as an initiate.

Womb Journey Meditation

You can either sit or lie down for this meditation as long as you are super comfy and won't be disturbed for 20 minutes or so. If you do not have a womb, ovaries or other organs, the energy of those organs will still be present in your body and available for you to use. Your womb space, or womb, lies deep in the body, just above the centre of the pubic bone, with the ovaries on either side, and a little behind it, but don't worry about the exact anatomy; this is an energetic exercise in exploring and building a relationship.

Let your eyes softly close, or lower your gaze if you prefer. Make yourself comfortable by dropping your shoulders and releasing the tension in your jaw. If it feels nice, place your hands over your lower abdomen.

Turning your attention inward, extend your next out-breath, and imagine that you are breathing out all the way down to your toes. As you breathe in again, breathe up your body from your toes up to the top of your head. Breathe down to your toes, and then breathe in up to the top of your head. Imagine or visualize how your breath creates a wave of relaxation that washes through you, releasing tension, softening your body. After a few more waves of relaxation, settle your attention in the area of your pelvic bowl.

Bring your awareness to the pubic bone at the front and centre of your pelvis. Imagine that you shrink yourself down and place your awareness inside your pelvis so that you can walk the perimeter and explore your pelvic landscape from the inside. Starting from the pubic bone, walk slowly clockwise towards your right hip, notice how strong and solid the bones are. You can imagine yourself stroking the bones as you go along. Admire your inner architecture, like walking around a historic place of worship. Notice the scars of your history and also your buoyancy and resilience. Continue your walk to the back of the pelvis where it meets the spine. Lean your hand up against the joints that contain you so strongly, while still allowing some flex. Continuing to your left hip, admiring the strength that the pelvic bowl provides you. Slowly, and with reverence, continue your walk to the front of the pelvis where we started. Notice the grounding your pelvis provides.

Now turn to face the features inside your pelvis. In the centre, your womb or, if you don't have a womb, the energy centre is still there as the centre of your creativity, giving you the magical ability to be born again, renewed every new moon. See your womb space full of light. If this space could speak, what might she say? If it feels right, listen to its message, however it arises and respond with love, if you can. If nothing arises, imagine giving her a hug.

Now come to your left fallopian tube and ovary, deep inside the body, centred above your hipbone, holding the feminine archetype for receiving, nurturing, gestating. See, feel or imagine it full of sparkling light.

Now move to your right fallopian tube and ovary, holding the masculine archetype for manifesting in the world, for roles and owning our creative capacity. Once again, imagine this right ovary full of light. Breathe love into both ovaries and fallopian tubes. Notice any images, feelings or sensations that arise.

Below your womb space, there's the cervix, a magical portal to your vagina. Send her some love, imagining her as a strong, responsive gateway.

Below the cervix is the vagina, which has the capacity to receive and also to protect you, another magical portal all to herself. Breathe into your vagina to support your capacity to root into the earth and stand steady in yourself. Then there's your vulva, beautifully unique and perfect just as you are. Hidden within, one of our greatest gifts, the clitoris, with thousands of nerve endings extending deep into the body. Give your attention and love to these magical places and ask them, 'What do you need to heal?' See what arises. If nothing comes, that's fine too; being open and asking the question is often more than enough.

Breathe the warm light of deep gratitude into your pelvic bowl, thanking it for the gifts that it brings.

It's time to draw the meditation to a close, so share any last words before you go. Now let your pelvic bowl fill again with warm light to wash away what you no longer need, and restore your centre. Take all the time you need to let this light wash you and release anything you no longer need; even if you don't quite know what that is, having the intention is enough.

It's time to make the return journey to everyday reality. Bring your awareness back to your breath once again, and as you breathe down to your toes, push your feet into the floor or give them a wiggle. As you breathe in, breathe up to the top of your head. Start to move your face, neck and shoulders in a way that feels good. Let your body move as you stretch your way back into the here and now. Softly opening your eyes, find a gesture to show yourself that the process is now closed.

After the meditation take a moment to write, draw or consider your experience. Were you surprised by what you found? By what was particularly alive, or absent? Is there anything you need to do to anchor what you have learned in your everyday life?

You can find a link to the audio for the Womb Journey Meditation on p. 392.

24 You are not alone

At any one time, a third of the world's female population are menopau-sal or postmenopausal. Think about it: that's 16 per cent of the global population who are potentially finding their power, using their voice, and getting ready to create change in their lives and communities right now! Far from being a crazy minority, we are becoming a force for change; for women to be heard, to educate the younger generation to use their voice. Do you think that the rest of the population might possibly be scared of this force for change? Maybe that's why there's so much negativity and shame around menopause. So, when you do feel like you're going mad, remember: you are most definitely not alone.

'IT WAS INSANELY EYE-OPENING FOR ME TO HEAR WOMEN FROM ALL OVER GOING THROUGH THE SAME THOUSAND THINGS AS ME, FROM PHYSICAL, EMOTIONAL, TO MENTAL. I STARTED WITH THE BOOKS ALREADY OUT THERE, AND I COULDN'T BELIEVE THERE REALLY WEREN'T ANY THAT NORMALIZED THIS EXPERIENCE.'

Kathleen

Listening partnerships

A listening partnership falls somewhere between counselling and having a loving friend with an objective view-point. They are a wonderful resource when you're going through the menopause and need a safe place to express difficult feelings, work out how you feel, or just take space to 'be'. It's an arrangement with a fellow menopauser where you can hold space for each other to be heard in confidentiality. In ordinary conversations between friends, there's often a dominant voice and conversation gets subverted by distractions, advice-giving and opinions. In a listening partnership, one person talks while the other actively listens without interrupting, offering their full attention. It's beautiful how the power of being heard in this way can give birth to understanding and insight. I was introduced to them at the leaderships training at Red School, but the concept was originally created by parenting organization Hand in Hand[1].

Guidelines for a listening partnership

- Find a partner – it can be an existing friend or a new one, just make it someone you trust.
- Find a venue that suits you both, such as Zoom, phone or in person.
- Agree on the boundaries: issues of confidentiality, timing, frequency, and anything else that might be important for you.
- Decide how long each of you will speak and who goes first.
- Share whether you prefer to be listened to in silence or if you'd like to hear any 'hmm's' or other responses to know you're heard.
- Before you start, take a moment or two of quiet to arrive in yourself.

THE LISTENER

- Sets a timer for the agreed time.
- Gives their attention to their partner and receives their words.
- Allows silence to be there if it comes.
- Tells their partner when the time is up and thanks them.

THE SPEAKER

- Can spend time just feeling into themselves and how they are.
- Can speak of anything that arises within them.
- Can ask for feedback afterwards if they would like it.

To keep the magic of the listening partnership, the things that are discussed in it are not talked about or referred to if you meet in a different situation or with anyone else.

PRACTICE

- Close your eyes for a moment, take a few breaths, now imagine all the menopausal women reaching out and holding hands across the globe. Feel the power of the connection and the force for good we are creating, let it flow into and through you.
- Find other menopausal women and create occasions to lean in and share your experience together, in a Red Tent, over coffee and cake, down the pub, a women's group maybe. If this doesn't exist, you can create a safe space to suit yourself and call in the people you want to be with.
- Create a listening partnership.

I am not alone in this experience.

25 Your body knows how to do this

If you are somewhere in menopause, your body will have made a similar transition around thirty-five years ago when you first had a period. You might have been angry, inarticulate, tired all the time, spotty, and feeling desperate. If any of this sounds familiar, it's no coincidence: both adolescence and menopause are times of unpredictable hormones, brain development and transition, and both are regarded with a degree of negativity in our society. Despite the difficulty, your body changed at adolescence without medication (unless you were put on the pill as a teen, but that's for another book) and it's also comes pre-designed to be able to make the change at menopause.

Your body knows how to do this. Just as the 14-year-old benefits from a kind, positive parent who nudges them to stay hydrated and get enough sleep, the menopausal you now needs your inner parent to guide you kindly to be gentle with yourself while your body does its work. Lynne Franks told me:

'I HAD A VERY EASY MENOPAUSE BECAUSE I HAD AN OUTDOOR LIFE; CYCLING, LOTS OF 5-RHYTHM DANCING, DRINKING LOADS OF WATER. I ALSO HAD A LOT OF BOYFRIENDS AND WAS LEARNING ABOUT MYSELF AS A SENSUAL WOMAN AND BEING IN MY BODY, WHICH WAS REALLY IMPORTANT.'

I often recommend to my clients that they imagine what their best friend would advise when they're troubled; it's a simple short cut to kindness and a loving relationship when we're stressed or down on ourselves. This can be particularly helpful is you have a disconnected or troubled relationship with your mum. You can also develop an avatar version of your inner self further to embody your intuition, inner wisdom or highest self or however you think about it by drawing, imagining and chatting with them. My inner wisdom is a little bit like me but sexier, braver, and with much better shoes.

PRACTICE

- Look at photos of yourself as a toddler and in your teens.
  Notice how that enormous shift in consciousness and physiology happened naturally.
- Imagine what advice your best friend would give you.
- Imagine or draw your higher self and see what advice she can give you.

My body knows how to do this!

26 Teenage kicks

Patterns naturally repeat in our lives. Themes return again and again, particularly those associated with major transitions such as birth, puberty, birthing babies and menopause. Themes from your birth and from the time of your first period are highly likely to surface for healing through your menopause years.

The way we are welcomed into the world has a profound effect on our experience[1]; my mum was put under a general anaesthetic when I was born, not unusual for Britain in the 1960s. The obstetrician had decided it would be better if she had a general anaesthetic as her hips were 'too narrow'. Goodness knows how my big sisters were squeezed out. The patterns of disconnection that this initiated have shown up in many areas of my own life, like anticipating that I would be left out of things, frequent numbing out, and finding intimacy a struggle. There was loneliness and no one around to support me when my period first came, repeating the theme. With awareness and self-kindness, I started to actively choose to be open to connection and to tolerate it more, and the loneliness that had dogged me through my life began to ease. Although the patterns may repeat, we are *not* the prisoner of our experiences, we *can* choose a different way.

Here's another story of how a client changed her patterns. After a surgical menopause, she reflected how she had been a caesarean baby herself and given birth to her babies 'through the sunroof' as she called it. There was a theme of rushed, unexpected interventions in her life; her life transitions tended to happen too fast, too soon, and her menopause too came on very suddenly. By consciously taking pauses in her day to breathe and feel what was happening in her body, she managed to become more present for herself, acknowledge how she was feeling, and regain a sense of pace and agency in her life.

What are the themes in your life?

It's interesting to reflect on the transitions in your life – your birth, your menarche, transfer to secondary school (which may well be bound up with your first period), house moves, divorces and pregnancies you might have had, or birthing experiences.

- What common themes can you find in these experiences?
- What challenges did you have?
- How was your journey through these events made easier or supported?
- What skills, talents or gifts have supported you in your transitions?
- How can you use these gifts and skills in your present situation?
- How can you bring small acts of kindness into your everyday life to bring healing to these patterns? This might be taking a breath, driving a different route, reaching out to a friend. See how creative you can be.

Exploring your first period, known as your 'menarche', the beginning of your Life Spring, has particular potency. Menarche is a time when we are particularly permeable to events happening around us. The way that we are received, how we feel about our gender, and the events going on around us can set the tone for how we feel about womanhood and femininity for the rest of our lives. This is especially true when we feel we don't fit the version of 'woman' that is presented to us as desirable, and when to be a woman at all is seen as problematic. It colours our experience of our menstrual cycle, fertility, motherhood, and menopause. Some people also believe that this is the time when our calling is sparked up and our direction in life. Whether you relate to this or not, it is an extraordinarily vulnerable time, when we're particularly permeable, and any trauma at this time will be played out through our lives.

'MY MUM NEVER SPOKE ABOUT
MENSTRUATION AND LETTING HER
KNOW ABOUT MY FIRST BLEED
WAS DIFFICULT. MAYBE IF I'D
HAD A CEREMONY I WOULDN'T BE
WORKING THROUGH SO MUCH INNER
CHILD/ADOLESCENT STUFF NOW IN
PERIMENOPAUSE, AND THOSE YEARS
WERE VULNERABLE AND MESSY.'

Nia

Some indigenous North American people believe that the dreams a girl has at this time give her a glimpse into her future life. Can you remember how dreamy you were as a teen? Even if you longed for something, anything, bigger and more expansive than your home life, that hope and opening into possibilities is so precious. The adoration of the latest, most beautiful, androgynous popstrel isn't about the person, or more likely, the team behind them, but about the rolling expanse of passion that an imagined future might contain. We're all familiar with how it feels when that bubble is burst and the hurt it brings to a tender young heart.

If you received positive messages about femininity and/or womanhood as a child, and you identify as a woman, then your process in menopause is likely to be considerably easier than if you have a negative view. If this is the case for you, taking time to heal the shame or wounding that occurred at menarche will ease your passage and let you move forward through menopause more easily. One way to do this is to hold a retrospective menarche ceremony where you can give yourself the particular welcome you would have liked to receive as a teen. Participants in our workshops are often surprised at how powerful it can be. It can be as simple or as elaborate as you like, with one friend or many. Don't be surprised, though, at how powerfully healing this can be, often in surprising ways. Here's an experience shared by women's health therapist Diane Przybilla:

> The biggest thing I got from the menarche ceremony was a total sense of who I am without attachments to any stories – strong, courageous and confident. In the months that have followed, I have felt a complete sense of freedom. Freedom to be the woman I was meant to be. I am also able to love, respect and honour my mother fully. In the past, in many situations, I would silently think to myself, 'Oh there we go, just like your mother.' My menarche ceremony brought the spiritual aspect of cutting the umbilical cord to life. It may have physically happened thirty-nine years ago, but I felt connected still. Only now do I feel that I am my own person entirely.[2]

PRACTICE
From the suggestions below, choose a way to reflect on your menarche and take steps to heal any wounds from that time.

- Reflect on the time around your first period: what was going on for you then?
- What were the messages you received about being a woman and about menstruation?
- Write a letter to your younger self, telling her everything she longed to hear at that time.
- Create a ritual to honour your first bleed and mark your transition. It can be as simple as lighting a candle or as richly complex as you'd like. You can find the names of people who will help you create a menarche ceremony in the Resources section.
- What pastimes, activities or inactivity did you love as a teen? How can you bring more of these into your life now?

I am so much more than the patterns in my life.

27 Meet the Autumn woman

If you are a woman who strongly identifies with her Inner Summer – the multitasking, sexy, capable, can-do person loved by all – menopause is going to be more psychologically challenging. It can be particularly tough if you get your self-worth mainly from being sexually attractive and look outward for other people to validate this. Of course, the Summer woman is the aspect that is highly approved of in our culture, so most of us, but not all, find it easier in this Season. As an Autumnal time of life, in Separation we are pulled out from can-do into can't-do and hopefully won't-bloody-do, and this is challenging if we feel our worth lies in doing things for others.

A woman who strongly identifies with her Autumn or Winter self will have developed more skills and tolerance of truth telling, resting, and letting go. She is more introverted perhaps and coming into menopause can feel like her natural home. Menstrual pioneer Rachael Crow told me:

'MY PERIMENOPAUSE AUTUMNS TAUGHT ME THE LESSON OF ACCEPTANCE AND SURRENDER. MY CYCLE WAS MY MAP AND WITHOUT IT I WAS FORCED TO STEP INTO TRUST. TRUSTING THE VOID, TRUSTING MY OWN INTUITION, ALLOWING MY INNER COMPASS TO GUIDE ME DEEPER INSIDE TO MY OWN WISE WOMAN TRUTH. NOW AS I STEP CLOSER TO BEING FULLY IN MOON PAUSE AND HOLDING MY WISE BLOOD INSIDE, I AM EXCITED TO BE FULLY STEPPING INTO THE PHASE OF ELDER. CROSSING THIS THRESHOLD CONSCIOUSLY WITH TENDERNESS AND SELF-LOVE, ALL THE WISDOM I HAVE GATHERED SUPPORTS ME. I TRUST THE PROCESS; I EMBRACE THE DEATH OF MY OLD FERTILE LIFE AS I LET GO AND STEP INTO THE NEW.'

You can see how practising menstrual cycle awareness offered Rachael a monthly glimpse into the void, so she was able to practise accessing the trust required to move consciously through her cycle. This means she can now apply the same trust to her menopause transition as she moves towards Second Spring.

PRACTICE

- If you still have a cycle, track your moods and energy through your menstrual month and reflect on which Seasons you feel most at home with and why.
- If you don't have a cycle, write down what you remember about your menstrual Autumn and Winter phases: what challenged you in these Seasons and what did you draw on to support you?
- You might like to use the Circle process (see pages 108–113) to re-visit the Seasons and gather information.

Learn to love the Autumn vibes.

28 Food and mood

You're glum, you're tired. What's the first thing you reach for? Comfort food obviously – *mmm*, that wonderful crusty white bread. But here's the bad news, refined carbs act as a kind of tranquilizer and can actually *trigger* mood swings, depression and fatigue. Your comfort food has quite literally become *discomfort* food. Suzanne Yates, the founder of Wellmother told me:

'I WAS EATING A HEALTHY SEMI-
VEGAN DIET, BUT FOUND I HAD
TO STOP DRINKING ALCOHOL,
EATING SUGAR AND GLUTEN,
THOUGH I RARELY HAD THEM
ANYWAY. I FELT CLOGGED UP
IF I DID AND THE RARE BRIEF
HOT FLUSHES, MORE A RASH ON
MY ELBOWS AND KNEES, WERE
AFTER I HAD TAKEN SOME OF THOSE.'

If bread isn't hitting the spot, how about something sugary – one of those adorable cupcakes as a pick-me-up? Nope. Sugar causes inflammation in the body, which means tissue damage and also insulin resistance. It will also contribute to fatigue, depression, anxiety, heart disease, and joint pain.

Damn it! No lovely bread and no sugar. OK, so let's have a glass of vino instead; didn't I read about the health benefits of red wine? And I am *so* much nicer when I've had a drink … Oh. Sorry. Firstly, alcohol slows the clearance of oestrogen by the liver, which can contribute to oestrogen dominance symptoms such as brain fog, sore boobs, sleep issues, hair loss, irritability, and depression. And it's high in sugar. And it affects the stress response system. Damn.

Fine, that leaves chips. I love chips, me. Well, potatoes are OK, but it's highly likely that they will have been fried in vegetable oil, which means they're coated in trans fats, which are so toxic they're banned in the US, having been linked to heart disease and obesity. So leave those chips alone.

You're knackered, right? That takeaway latte looks like a gift from heaven because it jump-starts our knackered body. However, coffee affects the blood-sugar function of the liver, so it can also cause hot flushes, increase stress levels, increase the risk of osteoporosis and, with deep irony, make insomnia and fatigue worse in the long term. It also decreases the availability of minerals and vitamins.

So. Bloody. Unfair.

Life is too short to eliminate the things we love. We've all experienced how if we restrict our food intake, we feel miserably deprived and crave the stuff we're not supposed to eat. Then we stuff our faces and hate ourselves for it; but it's not us that are broken, it's the diet fallacy.[1] Repeating an endless cycle of dieting and self-hatred is physically and emotionally damaging. If we can deal more effectively with our emotions by feeling them, instead of eating to stuff them down, we could eat what we want when we're genuinely hungry. 'A little of what you fancy does you good', as the old song goes, but if you're suffering, you could try cutting down or eliminating one thing to see if it makes a difference. Small lifestyle changes are the easiest to maintain; look at all those broken New Year resolutions when you go too hard all at once. Take a look at chapter 52 for inspiration on implementing workable changes into your life. Aim small – the little things all add up, I promise.

'I USED TO BE ABLE TO LIVE ON CARBS AND DAIRY. NO MORE. THEY DON'T LOVE MY BODY, NOT JUST FOR WEIGHT, BUT FOR ACHY JOINTS AND BLOATING. MORE PROTEIN, MORE FRUITS AND VEG. LESS STARCHES.'

Liz

For lots of us, it's a source of endless misery that our body fat is on the move and has taken up residence on our waists. To make it even more of an insult, no matter how well we eat and how much we exercise, it just doesn't seem to make any difference. Claire shares a familiar scenario:

When the anxiety moved in, my weight went haywire. It became a vicious circle of worry and weight gain. I started a new job = more stress = more weight gain. I was limiting my food more and more and still getting bigger. The irony is that now I've been home for six weeks, my body has been releasing and letting go. I'm noticeably different.

Some weight gain is inevitable, though; it's unrealistic to expect to be the size you were at 18. In fact doctors reckon that a realistic weight gain for a midlife woman is generally 10 kgs/22 lbs more than you weighed at 18. However, the change in hormone levels in midlife can trigger our poor, long-suffering nervous systems, leaving them strung out. Added to this, we've become used to living with 24/7 constant stress in our lives – and these stresses directly contribute to your muffin top. This is because both high *and* low levels of oestrogen are associated with fat gain around our middles, and these fluctuations also affect the hormones that regulate appetite. Add stress to the mix and our Stone Age nervous system misinterprets this as needing to lay down fat stores, because we're about to run from a sabre-toothed tiger any minute and will need easily available energy to do this.

'SWEETS. ALL. THE. TIME.'

Liz

We feel hungry for sweet things all the time. And hating yourself for being out of control/lazy/ugly, or whatever nasties your inner critic throws at you, just makes you more stressed. Limiting the calories we eat worsens the problem, because our over-sensitized bodies interpret this as a further stress factor. Then add in high intensity exercise, as often recommended, and the metabolism slows down even further because our body feels this is yet *another* emergency situation. You can change your diet and exercise like a maniac, but that beautiful, soft belly is not going to shift until you find ways to reduce the stress in your life and reset your nervous system. It's another case of the old ways of managing your life just not working anymore and a cry for more kindness.

> *I lay my hands*
> *on my beautiful hills*
> *I whisper soft mantras*
> *I whisper*
> *soft*
> *soften*
> *round*
> *juicy*
> *bloom*
> *I whisper*
> *take all the space*
> *you need*
>
> Clare Jasmine Beloved, 'Full Moon Belly'[2]

Now for the good news. Once your oestrogen levels become stable in Second Spring, anecdotally it seems that your body relaxes its vigilance and the belly fat seems to reduce *as long as you continue to eat well*. In short, don't give up, Second Spring is on its way!

PRACTICE

- Practise the Self-Care Abdominal Massage to connect with your belly, reduce stress and find what nourishes you from the inside (see pages 74–76).
- Love your liver: having a healthy liver function will help you manage your blood sugar and regulate hormones. Your liver loves lots of broccoli, leafy green veggies, garlic, onions, eggs, and mushrooms in your meals.
- Try castor oil packs to stimulate the lymphatic and circulation while supporting detoxification (see page 47).
- Buy bigger clothes – a beautiful way to prioritize your self-care. For silk kaftans, eBay is your friend.
- Notice what kind of foods you are craving and ponder on what feelings you might be trying to manage by eating them.

Feel the feelings, that's what they're there for.

29 Eat well, feel well

Confession time. I have always hated being advised about what to eat. It seemed to be delivered with a portion of smugness and a dollop of know-it-all that ignited my inner toddler and drove me straight to the doughnuts. Then in my Separation years something weird started to happen. My body started to crave green stuff; I asked for extra spinach in restaurants and craved more avocado. It didn't stop me from eating all the comfort food I loved; instead, it just started to tip the balance towards more nourishing options.

'CHANGES IN MY DIET HAVE BEEN
PROFOUND IN HELPING WITH ENDO
AND PERIMENOPAUSE SYMPTOMS.'

Nia

So I am not bossing you into bleeding all the pleasure out of your life, but inviting you to add in a little more of the good stuff that will help to balance hormones and feed your gut bacteria. Here's an overview:

Veggies: eating a rainbow is not a whimsical thing to do; it ensures you get the biggest range of nutrients possible. Cruciferous veggies such as broccoli and spring greens are especially good because they contain glucosinolates, which help to metabolize oestrogen.

Good fats: hormones are made from fats and cholesterol, and without enough 'good' fats, hormone production will suffer. 'Good' means the kinds of fats found in avocados, olive oil, coconut oil, and oily fish. These fats also help with the absorption of fat-soluble vitamins such as A, D, E, and K. Nutrient deficiency can often cause a hormonal imbalance, so not getting enough fat could be the cause.

Phytoestrogens: these are a special group of nutrients that are adaptogens, helping the body counteract and adapt to stress, which means they are handy when you're experiencing high or lower oestrogen. You can find them in nuts, seeds, whole grains, and legumes. A special place in heaven should be reserved for phytoestrogen-rich flax seeds and sesame seeds, which are your new best friends.

Sprouted seeds: from good old-fashioned mustard and cress to mung beans and alfalfa, phyto-oestrogenic sprouts multitask for you. They have fibre, feed your gut bacteria, help to eliminate toxins, and contain complex vitamins and antioxidants, as well as an impressive enzyme content. Sally Duffell's wonderful *Grow Your Own HRT* gives you the whole story.[1] Sow some cress on a bit of kitchen paper, right now!

Soy: the research is mixed on soy, but as unprocessed soy contains phytoestrogens it's often recommended. Take care to introduce these gently to your diet as if you eat a lot suddenly, they can create digestive problems. See if their presence makes you feel good. Try miso, edamame beans, or a little tofu.

Pleasure: the most life-changing ingredient to add to your meals is vitamin P—pleasure. Eating slowly and with pleasure has been shown to transform metabolic rate and assist the absorption of nutrients. So you might get more nutrition from a slice of cake eaten slowly than choking down a kale smoothie. Life is too short to force ourselves to eat stuff we hate.

Timing: managing your blood sugar well can really help with mood swings, especially anxiety; carry a little bag of nuts or a piece of fruit with you on your travels.

'CHANGING MY DIET HAS BEEN A STRUGGLE, ESPECIALLY TRYING NOT TO FALL BACK INTO OLD PATTERNS WHEN I'M LOW OR KNACKERED. BUT MY BODY SCREECHES OUT AT ME WHEN THIS HAPPENS, IT TRULY HAS HAD ENOUGH OF ME COCKING THINGS UP, AND MY DIGESTIVE SYSTEM SO LOVES IT WHEN I MAKE GOOD CHOICES. IT'S BEEN YEARS IN THE MAKING BUT EATING WELL BRINGS SO MUCH PEACE PHYSICALLY AND MENTALLY I WISH I HAD DONE IT EARLIER.'

Kate

It's important to remember that we all need different timing for our food: some people feel fabulous when they're fasting, but it turns me, for example, as crazy as a box of frogs. I'm more like a Labrador and need rhythm and regular pacing for my food. You probably already know what suits you and can rely on your own understanding of your needs.

Gut bacteria

Our guts contain about 3 lb of bacteria. Trillions of them make up our own unique microbiome; a world that is only just being explored. Recent research shows how gut flora influences our brain function, immunity, metabolism, mental health, stress response, and weight, and practically every other aspect of being human. It plays an important role in synthesizing B vitamins, which are essential for reducing fatigue, the risk of heart disease and for alleviating stress and anxiety symptoms. Your guts even hold the secret to happiness, as most of your serotonin is created in the cells lining the digestive tract.

We need to nourish our gut flora, and if you take good care of your microbiome during menopause, you can reduce symptoms.[2] Here's what your gut flora likes to eat:

Fibre-rich foods: a wide range of pulses, oats, nuts and seeds, veggies.

Prebiotics: these give your gut flora their favourite nosh; try garlic, onions, bananas, artichokes, and pulses. Also, one of my all-time favourites – potato salad, what bliss!

Probiotics: foods that contain live bacteria to help replenish your flora population, such as live yoghurt, kefir, sauerkraut, kimchi or kombucha. (What my family refer to as 'Mum's weird food', but wow, do they notice when I don't eat it!)

Inflammation

You'll be familiar with the kind of inflammation that happens when you sprain your ankle or get bitten by an insect. This acute inflammation is part of your body's healing response. Chronic inflammation, however, is when either your immune system doesn't turn off once its task is done, or it gets constantly triggered into action. It's particularly relevant at menopause, because one of the things that triggers inflammation is a lowered oestrogen level.

If you experience joint pain, increased belly fat, fatigue or brain fog, then inflammation may be playing a part. Your doctor can measure your level of C-reactive protein, a marker for inflammation, to see if chronic inflammation might be contributing to your problems. But there are also other clues to spot chronic inflammation:

- High blood glucose levels, which might show up as being thirsty, weeing a lot, having a dry mouth, and fatigue.
- Charming digestive issues such as gas, diarrhoea, bloating or constipation because of permeability in the gut walls.
- Skin issues such as eczema or psoriasis, or blotchy red patches.
- The runny nose and watery eyes brought on by allergies can be another indicator of inflammation.
- Gum disease, very common during menopause, can be a clue.
- Having a puffy under-eye area or face.

Long-term effects can include cardiovascular disease, diabetes, and osteoporosis, but the good news is that you can reduce inflammation with lifestyle changes:

- Reduce stress – yes, that again.
- Eat lots of fruit and veggies, especially dark-green leafy ones.
- Eat more 'good' fats like those in olive oil and avocados.
- Cut the crap – reduce sugar and refined carbohydrates.
- Eat bone broth: it contains the anti-inflammatory amino acids glycine and proline.
- Eat delicious food! There are lots of store cupboard herbs and spices you can add into your cooking to help reduce inflammation; turmeric, ginger, cayenne pepper, cinnamon, cloves, pepper and sage are all easy to use regularly in the food you cook.[3]

Changing your diet is notoriously hard and totally revolutionizing your diet is never sustainable in the long term. Instead make one small, do-able change at a time.

PRACTICE

- Choose one thing to add into your diet this week that will nourish you.

Choose pleasure!

Super-food with a Sting

When we're in a panic about our health, the combination of brain fog and Google makes it horribly easy to outsource our health solutions. Conveniently, there are people out there who would love to receive your money in return for fixing your 'oestrogen deficiency'. So instead of outsourcing, how about insourcing? There's a fabulously powerful, safe menopause remedy that is growing within walking distance of you right now – the humble stinging nettle (*Urtica dioica*).

If you're reading this in the dead of winter, or nettles don't grow in your area, you can buy them ready dried from your herb supplier and start from the fourth step, below. Nettle is a traditional herbal remedy used as a tonic to strengthen and support the entire body, and the high nutritional value makes them great for treating exhaustion, detoxing, strengthening the bones, alleviating joint pain, balancing blood sugar, strengthening the adrenals and kidneys, reducing inflammation, and managing stress. Their superpowers are due to their high level of nutrients, including vitamins A, B C and K, magnesium, phosphorus, potassium and zinc[1]. And they're free. The only sting in the tail is the sting!

WHAT TO DO WITH NETTLES

Pick the young shoots with gloves from a site situated well away from traffic or pollution. Give the nettle shoots a good wash before using.

Use them in cooking to make a soup or add to dishes as you would use spinach or greens. To make a nettle infusion:

- Wash and pat dry your fresh nettles.
- Layer your nettles with kitchen paper in a microwave.
- Process for 1 minute, and check them for crispiness, then process for 30 seconds at a time until they're dry but not cooked.
- Put 1 cup of dried nettles in a mason jar, and fill with 2 pints (1 litre) of boiled water.
- Leave the jar overnight.
- Strain and discard the nettles in your compost.
- Warm the infusion and drink hot straight away, or add ice. Keep cold in the fridge for up to 3 days.

Warning! The side effects may include thick, shiny hair, soft skin, and incredible *joie de vivre*. You have been warned.

30 Our culture makes it worse

So much for what we consciously put inside our bodies by way of food and drink; we also absorb the outer environment of our culture, which is sometimes quite toxic. The sophisticated mixture of fear of ageing shaken together with sexism creates a potent cocktail of negativity that impacts all of us. As we've touched on earlier in these pages, we are made to feel we are not good enough, that we have failed and/or should feel shame about ageing. Which of course makes for an enormous profit for the pharmaceutical and beauty industries.

Quite simply, we have been sold a lie to profit others and keep us under control in a mass cultural act of gaslighting. The widely used term 'ovarian deficiency' implies that we are somehow at fault for living beyond 50; there is no equivalent 'testosterone deficiency' spoken about in men. Patriarchy has painted menopause as a death, a passage into uselessness and decay that marks us as malfunctioning. I believe that this is partly because it's at menopause that the scales fall from our eyes and we rebel from patriarchal norms about how we should behave.

All this fear creates more stress, more rigidity, more isolation, and shame – which has been shown to make our symptoms worse[1] and maybe hold us back from being the person we aspire to be. If we decided that we truly liked our savoury selves and stopped buying into the saccharine, fear-based marketing that sells most cosmetics, we would actually be depleting the pockets of CEOs and shareholders. Whether it's dressed up as 'because you're worth it' or 'real beauty', the gaslighting that cosmetic companies use to sell us products is insanely profitable. The US cosmetic industry made a revenue of $54.89 billion in 2017, equivalent to the GDP of Croatia.

Once the scales have fallen from our eyes, there's no going back. However, we identify our gender, we are now able to define for ourselves what femininity means to us and which aspects of it, if any, we would like to embody, and to clearly discern what nourishes us, and reject the rest. As Dorothy Sayers says in *Clouds of Witness*:

'An advanced old woman is uncontrollable by any earthly force.'[2]

Cultural descriptions of older women are telling: wrinkled, dried up, harridan, used up, worn out, middle-aged old bag, harpy, crone, witch, saggy, heading south, letting herself go … Do you imagine that the patriarchy might, just possibly, be afraid of the power of older women? Even Twitter can seem medieval, as historian Mary Beard discovered:

> *'I get called a witch, often when I open my mouth to say something that the recipient doesn't like.'*[3]

Managing our contact with a toxic, ageist culture can become a highly nourishing superpower. You might choose to reduce or cut out social media, particular publications, TV or radio from your life. Even taking a short break can be very refreshing.

What if, as a wise client once suggested, the drying-up process was not a manifestation of our malfunctioning body, but instead, a process of concentration, like simmering a sauce down to its deepest, most intense flavours? A sweet plum becoming rich with flavour and depth? In the menopause process, our essence is revealed to us and it is deeply delicious. As oestrogen departs, the veil of caring, smoothing over, looking presentable, holding it together, not telling the truth, and putting others first has finally lifted. Menopause is the station where we can finally get off the train. We can stop judging ourselves by how others see us and prioritize our own pleasure.

'THE OESTROGENIC VEILS ARE LIFTED!'

Jane Hardwicke Collings, Women's Mysteries teacher

Far better then, to sideline a woman in her power as a witch; to marginal-ize, sneer at and discard this fearless, uncontrollable creature, *who will no longer put others' needs before her own and will continue to state the uncomfortable truth.* Far from being dried up, a woman in the Second Spring of her postmenopausal life has access to the well-spring of her creativity and self-love to be the change she longs to see, maybe even *because* of her reduced oestrogen! All over the world, there are hundreds of thousands of joyous postmenopausal women doing amazing things with their lives, finally the heroines of their own stories.

If we have our health and live to a ripe age, we are extremely fortunate. Women have never had as many opportunities and freedoms as we do now. If we get super lucky, we get to be an old woman; how cool is that?

PRACTICE

Here are some prompts to inspire enquiry:

- How might you reduce toxic media in your life?
- What thoughts or images come to mind when you hear the words 'old woman'? Are they useful for you to have?
- If there are any beliefs or attributes you hold about being an older woman that don't serve you? Where did they come from?
- Create a ritual to release any beliefs about ageing you don't wish to carry forward. You could write them down and burn, bury or flush them away. Sing them, shake them or stamp them out of your body.

I am the hero of my own journey.

31 Environmental damage

Besides the cultural toxins that we absorb, there are other harmful substances that we may take in from our environment. There is an enormous amount of evidence to show that chemical oestrogens, or 'hormone disrupting compounds' (aka HDCs), interfere with our hormones. The research is usually into their effects on fertility rather than menopause, because who wants to pour money into women's health if it doesn't result in babies, right? The evidence shows time and again how these hormone disruptors, in low doses over a long period of time, can cause earlier menopause and other oestrogen-imbalance problems. The main culprits are synthetic oestrogens in food, plastics, cosmetics, cleaning products, and water.[1]

Food

The synthetic hormones in food are found in factory-farmed meat, dairy, and as pesticides. The EU has banned the use of growth hormones in the animals we eat. The easiest way to avoid pesticides is to buy organic food where possible and wash your fruit and veggies before eating them.

Plastics

Plastics that contain Bisphenol A (BPA) are controversial.[2] Many manufacturers market their products as BPA-free and some countries have banned them altogether for their toxicity. There is also research that shows they are *not* a risk at low doses. You have to decide on the risk you are willing to take. Plastic labelled 'food grade' is monitored carefully for toxicity so you can enjoy that takeaway; however, microwaving your left-overs in plastic containers that are not labelled 'microwave safe' can leak dangerous phthalates (chemicals used to make plastic more durable), as can cling film in the microwave if it touches the food. Food from scratched or damaged plastic containers can also contain phthalates, so they have to be chucked into the recycling – which is not good for the planet or for you. I was gutted to find that most tins of food also have BPAs and that non-BPA-lined tins are stupidly expensive. Till receipts also have phthalates in them, who knew?

Cosmetics

My mum used to have a pot of Pond's Cold Cream that she used night and morning, and this was the extent of her skincare routine. The average 21st-century woman now uses about ten products each day, exposing herself to 515 chemicals every day. About 60 per cent of what we put on our skin is absorbed into our systems, most of which we have *no clue* about what it is. Parabens are particularly evil, increasing the risk of breast cancer. Look carefully at the ingredients for anything that ends in 'paraben', though hydroxybenzoid acid and hydroxybenzate are also nasties. There's an up-to-date list of paraben-free cosmetic companies at the Breast Cancer Action website.[3]

Cleaning products

The ads for cleaning products use their strength as a selling point, but they are more reticent when it comes to telling us how they might affect our health. In practice, the ingredients are not printed on mainstream cleaning products so if you are interested in balancing your hormones it's better to use an 'eco' brand that is transparent about what their products contain, or go old-style with vinegar and bicarbonate of soda.[4] Still not convinced? According to the World Health Organization:

> *The evidence clearly [shows] that industrial chemicals interfere with hormone action in ways that cannot be considered similar to natural environmental stressors and are often irreversible.*[5]

PRACTICE
- Buy organic and/or wash your fruit and veggies before use.
- Take your own glass or metal containers to the takeaway or only buy from restaurants that use paper containers.
- Check that plastic is microwave-safe and use a plate rather than cling film to cover food in your microwave.
- Clear out the cupboard under your sink and research homemade cleaning solutions.
- Filter your water with a filter jug or install a filter for your home if you can afford to.

I define myself by who I am, not what I do.

32 You will be hotter

Hot flushes are one of the most common experiences of perimenopause and menopause in the Western world. They can vary from a quiet glow to changing drenched sheets five times a night. Though commonly blamed on falling oestrogen levels, studies have also shown that the severity of flushes bear *no* relationship to the levels of oestrogen found in the body; in fact, the causes of hot flushes are still not properly understood.[1] Astonishing when so many are suffering, but as we already know, menopause health does not attract the research funding – it's just not sexy enough. What the researchers have found, however, is that activity in the central noradrenergic system *does* vary with flushes. Interestingly, this part of the brain also manages some aspects of the stress response. Flushing tends to be more frequent around the end of menstruation and tail off in Second Spring, though hot flushes can persist for a decade or more.

'I HAVE BEEN VERY SURPRISED AT HOW INTENSE HOT FLUSHES ARE. I THOUGHT IT WAS JUST A LITTLE BIT OF HEAT AND RED FLUSHING. IN REALITY, IT FEELS LIKE THE HIGHEST FEVER I HAVE EVER HAD, COMBINED WITH SUNBURN AND DEHYDRATION. WHAT I STRUGGLE WITH THE MOST IS IN THE MOMENT THAT IT IS HAPPENING, THERE IS NOT MUCH I CAN DO EXCEPT ACCEPT IT, AND LET IT HAPPEN. THAT'S VERY FRUSTRATING AND DIFFICULT TO NOT PANIC.'

Sharon

The first step to manage hot flushes is to chart when they happen and to notice what's going on when they do. Everyone has different triggers and understanding your own vulnerabilities empowers you to take care of yourself more tenderly. Possible triggers might include alcohol, sugary food, coffee, particular kinds of stress, thoughts and feelings, or relationship dynamics. Once you start to get a clear picture of what your triggers are, you can make informed choices.

Reducing stress will improve nearly all physical issues, so cutting out or delegating stressful tasks will help, and you can also try adding in meditative practices to your routine. Breathing at a pace of inhaling for five seconds and exhaling for five seconds, with your belly moving as you go, will calm the nervous system[2] and has been shown to reduce flushes[3].

Your mindset makes a massive difference. One woman shared how when she flushed, she pictured a fire-breathing phoenix awaking in her womb space, her power waking up. Another woman spoke of how she felt her flushes were like birth contractions, each one taking her closer to meet herself. If you can give a positive spin to your flushes, they will be more tolerable and less of an inconvenience. In Chinese medicine and homeopathy, energy is said to move towards the surface of the body to be released, so seeing the flush as a mechanism for letting-go can also be a powerful practice. As Dr Christiane Northrup explains:

> *Your beliefs and thoughts are wired into your biology. They become your cells, tissues, and organs. There's no supplement, no diet, no medicine, and no exercise regimen that can compare with the power of your thoughts and beliefs. That's the very first place you need to look when anything goes wrong with your body.*[4]

If you want to use complementary medicine, herbs or acupuncture are a good place to start. Herbal remedies are easily available or grown. Sage (although avoid this herb if you have a history of seizures) and black cohosh (similarly, don't use if you have a history of liver disorders) are effective for many people. Evening Primrose oil has been shown to reduce the frequency and severity of hot flushes, and also to even out mood swings and increase libido.[5] St John's Wort can work to manage flushes, but may interact badly with other medication such as contraceptives, anti-depressants or sleeping pills and make you prone to sunburn. Do your research carefully first.

If herbs aren't your thing, simply adding foods to your diet such as linseed, tofu, tempeh, miso, pumpkin seeds, sesame seeds or sunflower seeds can help to manage oestrogen levels. Eating oily fish and vitamin B6 have likewise been shown to reduce the severity of flushes.[6]

Where flushes are debilitating, HRT is a great option and can transform your life, so do speak to your doctor about your options.

PRACTICE

- Keep a diary or use a lunar chart (see chapter 51) or menstrual cycle chart (see chapter 6) to note your flushes and what triggers them. Once you've identified your triggers, what changes could you make to reduce the impact of your flushing?
- To use the flushes as a tool for growth, try using these journaling prompts and free-write for 10 minutes; you might be surprised at what emerges:
  - 'What is it that wants to be released here?'
  - 'What is it that needs my attention?'
  - Take a moment to be comfortable in yourself, whether standing or sitting with your spine lengthened, and roll your shoulders back a few times on your out-breath. Yawn a bit to relax your jaw. Either counting or using a timer, breathe in for 5 seconds and out for 5 seconds. If this is comfortable, you can extend it to 6 seconds. You can do this as part of your meditative practice or even when washing up.

Your wisdom is rising. Rise, sister, rise!

33 Tame your inner critic

Self-awareness is the gateway to wellbeing, but studies show that non-judgement is Queen, and it's the strongest predictor of wellbeing. In a study looking at the role of mindfulness on anxiety, the people who weren't so judgemental of themselves were less impacted by their symptoms. To put it the other way, judging yourself worsens your symptoms, making you doubly miserable.

Knowing about the phases of menopause and how we release the old before we welcome the new is a great help. But often as soon as the idea of releasing the old arises, your inner critic shows up. Sometimes she's clearly audible: 'You're pathetic to be feeling so low, just get on with it, you should have handled it by now!' (A favourite of mine.) But sometimes she is sly to the point of being undetectable and we have ingested 'you are shit' for so long we cannot see it as an external force; it's become an integrated part of ourselves.

'I BELIEVE THAT THOSE NEGATIVE SELF-BELIEFS ARE INTROJECTED INTO US FROM KEY AUTHORITY FIGURES IN OUR LIVES AT AN EARLY AGE. TO BREAK "THE RULES" TAKES SOME UNDOING, DEPENDING ON THE RELATIONSHIP WITH THE AUTHORITY FIGURE, AND UNTIL WE HAVE SOMETHING BETTER TO REPLACE IT WITH, INTROJECTS ARE OFTEN STILL USEFUL TO US, HOWEVER PERVERSE THEY SEEM. A BIG PART OF THE WORK IS LEARNING WHAT THESE INTROJECTS ARE AND HOW THEY'RE STILL HELPFUL TO US. ONLY THEN CAN WE REALLY CHOOSE A DIFFERENT BELIEF OR RULE FOR OURSELVES.'

Emily Sugarman, Gestalt psychotherapist

Sometimes it takes a kind friend or therapist to point out that this or that belief is not a fact, but actually part of a toxic inner critic.

Have you ever noticed how that we chuck out the compliments with the trash but clutch hold of criticism like jewels? It seems perverse, but it's part of our primitive survival mechanism; our Stone Age selves are never far from the surface. Luckily, it's not a fixed state, because our brains have neuroplasticity and our wiring is adaptive. Neuroplasticity explains why the things we do most often are what we become stronger at, while what we don't do fades away. This is why repeating a thought or action increases its power. After a while, it's automated and we literally become what we think and do.

'THE MORE WE STAY IN THE NEGATIVE STRESS RESPONSE, THE MORE WE LAY DOWN SYNAPSES THAT TAKE US QUICKLY INTO THAT SPACE. SO, IT BECOMES NORMAL TO QUICKLY FIND OURSELVES IN DRAMA OR ANGER OR TANTRUMS OR ANXIETY. IT TAKES TIME TO LAY DOWN NEW SYNAPSE PATHWAYS SO THAT OUR DEFAULT RESPONSE IS LESS NEGATIVE. ALSO, THIS IS SUPER EASY WHEN WE ARE CHILDREN BUT SLOWS DOWN IN ADULTHOOD.'

Melonie Syrett, menstrual health educator

In other words, we need to put in a little energy to loosen our inner critic's grip so she doesn't have us so tightly clamped in her jaws that we cannot breathe at all; *then* we can lay down new neural pathways for a different way of thinking. The critic's natural home is in the Autumn, your premenstrual phase and perimenopause, so she typically shows up here shouting loud and clear.

But there is gold in them there hills; your critic does have valuable things to contribute to your life. Red School, the trailblazing menstrual and menopause educator, teaches that the inner critic has a 'sacred role' in awakening us to a new level of power by pricking our egos, helping us to address our shadow side, and to midwife our calling into life. Sounds unlikely doesn't it? But my friend and colleague Leora Leboff explains how it can look in real life:

When I engage with my inner critic and see her as a separate part of myself, I can shine humanity on her words. Every time she dumps on my worth the kinder part of me can have a sensible conversation with her hatefulness. Although she delivers words unkindly, there's always something useful to be heard as well. The kinder voice unearths the treasure hidden in the shit.

So, the inner critic is worth paying attention to. If you struggle with your critic and you are still menstruating, I can strongly recommend the chapter on the inner critic in Red School's book *Wild Power*.[1] What follows are some alternative ways of thinking to at least get some wiggle room and at best harness the creative force of your inner critic.

It's not your fault

Each wound has a seasonal cycle all to itself, growing louder and quieter by turns, offering us more information about our inner critic each time. When you become aware of yours it is not because you haven't 'done your work' or 'got it right'; it's because being cyclical is what cycles do. We tend to make everything *so* much harder by judging ourselves for the arrival of the issue to begin with, even before we deal with the matter. Here are some things to consider:

- We would like to be 'healed' in a one-stop shot, but in real life, the same themes show themselves periodically, revealing deeper layers of meaning. It's OK; you're OK.
- Feelings come in cycles, becoming intense and then easing off – but feeling the emotion doesn't trap you in it. The energy of the cycle has an intelligence that wants to help you move through it. It may hurt like hell but it's not mortally dangerous: 'all' you need do is allow it for a while before it shifts.
- Feelings are as natural as pee and poo. You don't tell yourself not to go; you just wait for the appropriate time to do it, somewhere safe and hopefully, clean enough.
- Just as you don't start with a heavy weight on your first trip to the gym, you need to build muscle when it comes to dealing with your beliefs and feelings. Being interested in some small issue without judging it is a great way to start. Don't charge into long withheld grief straight away and expect to feel neutral.
- Our critics often have a huge desire to keep us safe from pain, it's just that they express their concern in horrible ways. They want us to stay small, keep safe and stay out of trouble.
- Instead of locking up the uncomfortable feeling in a box like it was an evil gremlin, imagine it was a baby human or a baby animal in need of warmth and safety.
- You are enough.

PRACTICE

When we are criticized, our natural impulse is to move far away from that horrible voice as fast as we can, but trying to shut down our inner critic and putting our fingers in our ears just makes them shout louder. In order to quieten them down, we need to build a relationship with them, to listen and respond. There are various ways you can experiment with doing this.

- Sometimes your inner critic may take the tone of real people in your life, so go ahead and name them.

- Even if they are not like an actual person that you can identify, it can sometimes be helpful to give them a name anyway. (Mine is called Piranha).

I am doing the best I can, and that is enough.

Ways to Manage Your Inner Critic

You can explore the critical voice with stream of conscious writing, by drawing or by having a dialogue with them. This is an exercise for when you are feeling relatively robust. If your mental health is vulnerable, delay this until you're feeling stronger.

Slow. Everything. Down. So that you can hear your inner critic. Breathe and go slow.

Make sure you have a nice snack available: low blood sugar is a killer.

Identify a specific criticism, write it down in your journal and respond. Try to focus on one specific criticism. Inner critics like to broaden the negativity to the point that you end up in a shit-storm and no dialogue is possible, so staying specific gives to you space to talk.

Having an imaginary friend/ best friend/superhero protector nearby can be really helpful now. Employ your protector superhero/best friend/ avatar to answer the critic's questions if you like, so you don't have to.

Be your own best friend too and take your side as you respond to what your inner critic says. There are many other imaginative ways you can deal with critics, such as by imagining sailing them away, gagging them, throwing them away, sinking them in jelly. Have fun and get creative with ways to lessen your own critic's power.

Afterwards it can be nice to return the paper on which you've written down your responses to the elements with a ritual burning, or by flushing it down the loo, or burying it. Even simple rituals can be very powerful.

Top tip: When your critics ambush you in daily life, say to yourself, 'That is my inner critic speaking'. Naming is a powerful tool that can give you more room to breathe.

34 Sense and sensitivity

'I'VE BECOME MORE SENSITIVE TO
NOISE. I WORK IN A BUSY OPEN-PLAN
OFFICE AND SPEND A LOT OF TIME ON
TELECONFERENCES. I FIND IT VERY HARD
TO HEAR WHAT PEOPLE ARE SAYING
WHEN THERE IS A LOT OF BACKGROUND
NOISE. I THOUGHT MY HEARING WAS
GOING, BUT IT'S FINE. I JUST CAN'T STAND
DIFFERENT NOISES AT THE SAME TIME.
WHEN MY SON AND HUSBAND BOTH TALK TO
ME AT THE SAME TIME ABOUT DIFFERENT
THINGS (WHICH HAPPENS A LOT) IT DRIVES
ME MAD. DON'T GET ME STARTED ON THE
SOUND OF PEOPLE EATING.'

'Holly'

Do you have teenagers in your house? Or perhaps you remember your own or your siblings' moodiness, needing to be alone, or behaviours that were clearly irrational in retrospect however passionate we felt at the time.

Despite the challenges of adolescence, we can hopefully bring kindness and gentle guidance to our young people, knowing that they'll grow out of it eventually and become fully functioning adults. Pregnant women are given the greatest consideration too while they grow a baby inside them, as they are also prone to fatigue and moodiness. Both pregnancy and adolescence are times of great hormonal upheaval where we are in an 'in-between' space between child and adult, between woman and mother.

In puberty, pregnancy, and menopause we're in between states, both in terms of our identity and our hormones – so we are way more sensitive. Sensitive to noise, stress, foods, more allergies, more emotional sensitivity, lies, bullshit: in all kinds of ways our skin is thinner, and we are more permeable.

'I CANNOT TOLERATE ANYTHING RELATED TO ANIMAL CRUELTY, AND I'M ALSO MORE SENSITIVE TO HUMAN SUFFERING. IT'S AS THOUGH I FEEL THE PAIN PHYSICALLY. MY ANGER HAIR-TRIGGER IS ALSO A BIT MORE READY TO BE PULLED AND IT IS WORSE DURING WEEKS FOUR AND ONE OF MY CYCLE.'

Emma

We become super sensitive; the combination of psychological development and hormonal shift means that we will be more sensitive both psychically and physically. In Separation particularly, we don't know where we are *at all*. All sorts of things that might have been shrugged off before now penetrate us more deeply. It's not only unkind words – previously unknown food sensitivities can become activated, some of us become hyper-sensitive to smells, bright lights or noise. We can be kind and caring to teens and pregnant women in their liminal state, but can we deliver the same generosity and understanding as we prepare to birth ourselves?

'I'VE BECOME SENSITIVE TO BLOODY EVERYTHING AROUND ME, LIKE EXPERIENCING A DIFFERENT STATE OF BEING. I'M ALSO SUPER SENSITIVE TO A WHOLE RANGE OF FOODS THAT HAVE ALWAYS BEEN A REGULAR PART OF MY DIET.'

Catherine

And then there is an increased sensitivity to stress.

'MY STRESS LEVELS HAVE BEEN
INSANE. IT JUST NEVER STOPS.
MY REACTION TO THINGS THAT
ARE STRESSFUL IS SO MUCH MORE
THAN EVER BEFORE. ON A PHYSICAL
LEVEL, I'M VERY STRESSED. I FEEL
MY EMOTIONAL UPSET AFFECTING
MY PHYSICAL SYMPTOMS MORE.
IT REALLY FEELS LIKE I'M NOT
MYSELF ANYMORE.'

Kathleen

By now you'll have got the message about the benefits of slowing down and managing your stress more effectively, and hopefully you'll have made a few changes in your life. But here's the thing – you need to put even *more* things in place, because menopause actually makes us more sensitive to stress. Just at the most challenging part of our lives too, when the combination of pushing on the glass ceilings, managing adolescents and ageing parents all at the same time makes for an 'interesting' time.

Here's an overview: oestrogen has a role in managing the levels of cortisol in the body, so as oestrogen levels fluctuate or drop, we're less able to regulate cortisol levels as effectively, and feel more stressed as a result. Also, the adrenal glands have a secondary function in producing oestrogen when the ovaries are slowing down, but those poor, knackered adrenals will always prioritize stress hormone first, so oestrogen drops further. And we feel more stressed.

'I THINK I WAS SENSITIVE ANYWAY, BUT I WOULD SAY THAT IN MENOPAUSE I CAN'T TOLERATE THINGS AT ALL, SO IT'S REALLY HELPED ME ADDRESS STRESS POINTS AND TAKE ACTION.'

Jessica

Listening to disabled people and those with pre-existing health conditions, I have heard many stories of existing health conditions being aggravated during these women's menopause. For example, I have spoken to women with diabetes who find it more difficult to keep blood sugar levels stable, and to others who struggle with symptoms of multiple sclerosis, or with their fibromyalgia being exacerbated. This is likely to do with the role that oestrogen plays throughout the body's systems, including sensitivity to pain. Menopausal symptoms may also be made worse by the disabled person's health condition, and it can be more difficult for a disabled woman to get the medical support they require, or to recognize the symptoms as being related to the menopause.

PRACTICE
- What one thing could you drop today? What could you delegate, reschedule, say no to, shove under the carpet ... just one thing?
- Make a wish list of any food, comfort, activity and rest you would love to have in your day. How could you give yourself 1 per cent of this?
- What can you commit to giving yourself today?

- Cross your arms in front of your body and soothe yourself, stroke or gently pat yourself.

Please be gentle with your sweet self.

35 Your brain is growing

'BRAIN FOG. WHAT A HORRIBLE FEELING THAT IS. FORGETTING HOW TO DO THINGS I'VE BEEN DOING FOR YEARS — LIKE HOW TO OPERATE THE PETROL PUMP AT THE SAME FILLING STATION I'VE USED FOR YEARS. SCARY!'

Sandra

Brain fog is a real thing.[1] Getting lost driving familiar routes, forgetting words, and having no clue why you're standing in a room. All familiar stuff, no doubt, and troublesome when you're trying to operate at work and manage a family. Brain fog is intertwined with sleep deprivation and stress, often creating a catch-22 of panic as we worry about how the hell we're going to cope.[2] If this wasn't disorientating enough, often the words to describe our experience go into hiding too. My colleague Leora Leboff puts it this way:

I see women who are able to say so much about their menopause. Yet sometimes my own words are gone. Part of the time I beat myself up, questioning why they've left me. Part of the time I'm wrapping myself in kindness and feeling those edges and all the discomfort. I also trust that one day, my words will come back.

Leora's right: they will come back once the hormonal swings have evened out and, no, you don't have dementia. It can be very frightening because our memory is so fundamental to our deep sense of self. Like in the film *Memento*, without it we are lost and our idea of who we are seems to be strung on a narrative thread of past events and planned action. The good news is it's not permanent and the fog clears in the years following your last period.

While short-term memory can be impaired through hormonal fluctuations, there is also something else happening: the part of the brain responsible for making judgements, solution finding and managing emotions is actually developing[3]. In our forties and fifties, we use more of our brain and become better at positive thinking and managing our emotions. We develop greater capacity to see patterns as we age: where younger people cannot see them, we can connect the dots from our lived experience to understand more of what is going on and what might happen next; we can see the bigger picture. Our brains may be slower than a 20-year old's but we are, biologically, wiser.

From a body–mind perspective, maybe our slower and foggier brains are signalling something connected with growth. They can be seen to be directing our attention away from the external world and give more importance to our emotional lives, reflecting on where we're at and how we want to be in the world. It's one of the ways our body brings us into Separation. According to Dr Christiane Northrup, our brains are being rewired to make this possible.[4] The high levels of follicle-stimulating hormone and luteinizing hormone present in menopause drive positive change in our brains, serving as extra neurotransmitters on the right side of brain. This increase optimizes creativity, intuition, and visionary experiences – the real juice of menopause. It's part of the physiology of Second Spring developing in our minds, preparing the way. There are also changes in the brain that help us perceive things more clearly. Another hormone, namely gonadotropin-releasing hormone or GnRH, which is the precursor to follicle-stimulating hormone, is priming the menopausal brain for new perceptions.[5]

Or how about this for a reframe: brain fog as the ultimate in mindfulness. Even neuroscientist Daniel Levitin speaks of this.[6] Not only does it bring you smack bang into the present (ouch), it also brings you the empty mind much longed for by meditators all over the world. Forgive me if once again I offer a male to female comparison; if cis men had brain fog it would be heralded as a consciousness breakthrough. For women, it's perceived as a breakdown. Or, how about when a 25-year-old forgets something and they reason that they've been carrying a lot in their life, so it's no wonder they forgot? The way we describe our forgetfulness can make the fog better or worse. The next time your mind is wiped in the middle of a conversation, you can say, 'Sorry, my mind is busy transforming my psyche, I can't meet your needs right now.' Better still, have it printed on a little card, like a 'Get out of jail free' card in Monopoly. There is no shame in mindfulness. Brain fog *can* be incapacitating at times, but it's not the whole picture.

PRACTICE
- Have a look at how you can improve the way you manage stress and choose a breath, meditation, mindfulness, or movement

practice to do every day that brings you into a calm space.

- Chart the severity of your brain fog and see if you can see what triggers you.
- Have a look at the suggestions for managing low oestrogen and/ or high cortisol in chapters 3 and 29.
- Lose control. Laughing at the sheer madness of it all is incredibly liberating.
- Try increasing your levels of B12 (a vitamin that helps to keep the body's nerve and blood cells healthy) by eating more meat, eggs and dairy or taking a B12 supplement.

Relax. Nothing is as important as you think.

36 Your sleep may suffer

You are very tired yet sleep eludes you. All you ever read is how the lack of sleep makes you ill and vulnerable, so you worry about that too, and then you can't sleep at all. There are many products that offer the promise of better sleep, but I'm going to stick my neck out here (on a supportive pillow) and say that none of them, by themselves, is going to fix your sleep. I wish they would, but they won't. What's going to help you is to use your awesome menopausal discernment to assess your sleep hygiene, identify what soothes you and how to re-establish your circadian rhythm. If you do this then eventually sleep will return.

'THE LACK OF SLEEP AT NIGHT IN THE DARK CAN BE LONELY AND OF COURSE YOUR BRAIN GOES EMOTIONALLY HAYWIRE THE FOLLOWING DAY. I'M EXHAUSTED MENTALLY AND PHYSICALLY. IT REALLY MESSES WITH MY DIABETES.'

Kate

It's interesting to note that getting eight hours' straight sleep is a relatively recent phenomenon[1]. Nirlipta Tuli of The Yoga Nidra Network explains that we are not biologically wired to sleep an eight-hour stretch and that in preindustrial society it was common to have two or more sleep phases.[2] This 'sentinel' sleeping pattern can still be seen in the Hadzas, hunter gatherers in Tanzania, who take it in turns to be on watch at night, and where, at any one time, about a quarter of the community are awake[3]. They might have a first sleep when it gets dark, then wake in the middle of the night to feed the baby or prepare the bread dough, followed by a second sleep until it is time to wake in the morning. The 'sentinel' sleep pattern positively affects their circadian rhythm, optimising their body processes, including the endocrine system[4].

In experiments, the night watch has been shown to be a time of relaxed attention and calm, far from the whirling storm of anxiety-riven insomnia[5]. It's wonderful to know that waking up at night is normal: it's not a pathology. There are also seasonal variations, with winter darkness bringing more hours of sleep and lighter summer nights requiring fewer. Translate this into women's menstrual cycles and there will likely be more sleep in the Autumn/premenstrual phases and Winter/period times and less around ovulation.

Sleep coach Nick Littlehales looks at the total number of sleep cycles over a week, including naps, to give his athlete clients an edge.[6] In short, we need to find our own sleep rhythm and know that this rhythm will also have seasonal variations. And that's OK. There is no one way to sleep that is 'correct' all the time, so you can relax about this at least. Like many menopausal symptoms, sleep issues usually melt away once you reach the calm hormonal seas of Second Spring.

'IT STARTED AROUND 42. WAKING UP IN THE NIGHT FOR A FEW HOURS THEN BEING EXHAUSTED. I'VE REALLY HAD TO SLIM DOWN MY LIFE. START WORK LATER, NOT WORK TOO MANY HOURS, WORK FROM HOME REGULARLY. LUCKILY, MY JOB IS VERY FLEXIBLE, BUT I'VE PROBABLY STAYED IN A JOB THAT I'VE OUTGROWN TOO LONG AS IT FITS ROUND MY ENERGY LEVELS.'

'Clare'

The question is not 'how well did I sleep?' but 'how well can I rest?' and be more like the Hadza?

Audit your sleep hygiene

You'll have read this advice a thousand times before, but are you actually doing it? It's worth taking a real-world sleep hygiene audit before you make further changes or spend money on pills:

- Avoid bright lights before bed time – and that includes screens!
- Sleep in a dark, cool room.
- Eat early and lightly in the evening.
- Get outside for some natural light in the morning.
- Take a gentle walk in the early evening.
- Avoid/reduce caffeine and alcohol.

PRACTICE
- Prepare for bed from the moment you wake up – look at your circadian rhythm and see what you can do to be more wakey-wakey in the morning and super soothing in the evening.
- Try Coherent Breathing®, which is breathing in and out for the same length of time. Using a timer or app, try 4 seconds in and 4 seconds out. If that feels comfortable you can lengthen the breath to 5 or 6 seconds. This switches on the relaxation response.[7] You can also explore using sleep tape to prevent mouth breathing at night; check out James Nestor's research in his book Breath: The New Science of a Lost Art.[8]
- Make a list of the things that soothe you:
  - Food: different types of food, pace and rhythm/quantity of meals.
  - Pace of life: space and structure of your free and working time (this took me years).

- Screen time and social media: what are helpful boundaries?
- Movement: what kind of movement, and what time of day is best?
- Connection: how much social time, where, doing what, how often, with whom?
- Pastimes: even those things we love can wind us up, so keep an eye on your pace, timing and obsessiveness!
- Naps: are they helpful for you? If so, for how long and when?

Do less. Then do less again.

37 You will shed identities

'I HAVE LET GO OF EVERY ROLE UTTERLY,
SOME I HAVE DROPPED, SOME I DO BETTER AND
SOME I HAVE CHANGED SO RADICALLY THAT
PEOPLE NO LONGER WANT TO INTERACT WITH ME.'

'Tanya'

In Separation, more than any other time in our life, we have the opportunity to declutter identities that no longer fit us. We may have adopted particular ways of being when we were girls – 'the kind friend' or 'the creative one' or 'the funny one' – because we were rewarded for them. Over time, we find it's easier to wear this mask than to express the often contradictory mix of strengths and vulnerabilities we feel. These masks have become hardened over time, and now, for us to be reborn through the menopause transition, they are cracking in preparation for being shed.

'*CAN'T BE ARSED* IS A MANTRA THAT SEEMED TO HAVE STUCK WITH ME. I DON'T NEED TO GET INVOLVED IN OTHER PEOPLES' DRAMA AND EXPECTATIONS OF WHAT I *SHOULD* BE. I LOVE THE FREEDOM THIS BRINGS.'

Kate

Sometimes letting go of a particular role feels like we have to let go of our entire identity – and our egos definitely don't like that. This brings to light a core aspect of menopause, in which, like any initiatory process, we have to let go of who we think we are. As far as our ego is concerned, we *do* have to die to move forward. Joseph Campbell, a Jungian-influenced professor of literature with a particular interest in myths, wrote about a process called the 'hero's journey' – an archetypal voyage of maturation that humans embark upon. In it, he describes this part of the initiation as 'the abyss', where we must die and be reborn. It's the Royal *The Grand Knockout Tournament* of 1987, Bowie's 'Laughing Gnome', or Madonna's 2019 Eurovision performance: identities were exposed as unworkable and it was clearly time for a rethink. Incidentally, Joseph Campbell was responsible for the wonderful phrase 'follow your bliss', which is an excellent path to lead you out of the abyss.

'EACH AND EVERY DAY I'M WORKING ON SHEDDING IDENTITIES. WHEN I FIRST STARTED THE PROCESS, I IMAGINED THAT I HAD LITTLE HOOKS IN THE FLESH OF MY LOWER BELLY AND I WAS SLOWLY UNHOOKING THEM, ONE BY ONE, HANDING BACK ROLES THAT I ONCE EMBRACED AND ENJOYED, BUT WAS NOW READY TO DROP OR SPREAD AMONGST THE REST OF THE FAMILY.'

Jessica

Another Jungian, Clarissa Pinkola Estés, author of *Women Who Run with the Wolves*, speaks of menopausal women 'hanging their skin on a spike in the underworld', which echoes Jessica's statement. Ouch.

'SECOND SPRING AND THE COVID PANDEMIC HAVE COMBINED TO GIVE ME THE CONFIDENCE AND IMPETUS TO UNHOOK FROM THE MAINSTREAM OF CORPORATE WORK AND CAREER TO FINALLY BE ABLE TO GIVE MYSELF A BREAK FROM BEING A WAGE EARNER, AND HAVE TIME TO LOOK AT MY NEEDS AND WANTS. TO HAVE THE TIME TO TAKE UP MORE INTERESTS AND HAVE TIME TO CARE FOR MYSELF AS WELL AS MY FAMILY, WHEREAS BEFORE IT WAS MY FAMILY'S NEEDS WHO ALWAYS GOT MET BEFORE MY OWN.'

Louise

For parents of older children, the empty nest means there's no role for the mother. Stress and anxiety make the 'big job' unendurable. These crunch moments bring us to the abyss where we're forced to shed the role and it feels *terrifying*, with our inner critic running rampant. Naturally, we move away from these challenging feelings, imagining that the emotion is going to cause us fatal damage, and instead spend lots of time and money trying to 'fix' the issue.

'I THINK I MIGHT GIVE UP
BEING A VIOLINIST AND
BECOME A NURSE INSTEAD.'

'Maggie'

Menopause requires us to lose it, to let go, to release. In one sense, these crises are Separation trying to move us into Surrender – where we can admit, finally, that in this liminal space we don't yet know who we are becoming. Menopause wants us to be all of who we are, to open up the possibilities so we can be helpful and withdrawn, a caregiver and an adventurer, a leader and vulnerable; losing our outgrown armour gives us the possibility of being bigger.

Being forced to let go of identities can feel like a death but often it's not the job that has to go, but the motivating force behind it: the desire to be seen as 'successful' or 'motherly' or 'competent' that hook into us. If we can heal the motivation behind the role, it may not mean we have to let go permanently. Nevertheless, we must be willing to make the commitment to ourselves by stepping into the unknown so we can grow up.

'IN SOME WAYS I FEEL LIKE I'M
BECOMING MORE MYSELF. AS
IF I HAD A "TOUGH GIRL" ACT GOING
MY WHOLE LIFE AND NOW I'M JUST
STANDING IN MY STRENGTH AND ALL
THE SENSITIVITY.'

Kathleen

PRACTICE

- Look out for times when you feel your mind and body starting to grip harder; this might show up as obsessive thinking, repetitive thoughts, 'shoulds' and 'musts', or fear in the body manifesting in the form of physical tension. When you spot these, give them love, treat them like you'd treat your best friend when she's upset or a hurt child. Love them. Hold them. Stroke them and give them the words you long to hear from your mother or your lover. This is your medicine.
- Breathe into the physical tension, allow it to be there and create softness around it.
- Where roles don't fit but it's hard to let them go, you could choose to 'shelve' them for a period of time and come back to review your situation on a particular date.

Use the Clearing Meditation to help you let go (see pages 54–56).

Follow your bliss.

38 No more babies

'NOT BEING ABLE TO HAVE CHILDREN IS
THE MOST DIFFICULT EXPERIENCE OF MY
LIFE. I HAVE COME A LONG WAY. I KNOW
NOW THAT I DON'T NEED A CHILD TO
HAVE A LIFE OF PURPOSE, BUT THE
DESIRE TO HAVE A CHILD — THAT NEVER
GOES AWAY. I'M NOT AS ASHAMED OF IT
AS I WAS AT FIRST.'

Lizzie Lowrie[1]

Today, in a culture where for millennia a woman's worth has been judged exclusively by the productivity of her womb, what the hell is the point of a menopausal woman? In a not-too-distant dystopian future, perhaps the likes of Trump and Boris Johnson and their ilk may well suggest a chemical termination, to save the bother of dealing with us. Back in the contemporary world, though, recent medical developments such as ovarian grafting might be able to delay menopause for twenty years or so, but there's no getting away from the truth that menopause brings an end to the possibility of having biological children. If you haven't had children, even though you may feel you've made peace with it already, a sense of loss can come up from under and knock you over, as you grieve for what was not to be.

'HAVING HAD YEARS OF PAIN WITH MY MENSTRUAL CYCLE, THE MENOPAUSE CAME AS SOMETHING OF A RELIEF, BUT ALSO A SURPRISING LOSS. I REMEMBER MISSING THE REGULAR RHYTHM OF THE CYCLE, AND MISSING MY BLEEDING ITSELF, EVIDENCE AND EXPERIENCE OF MY WOMANHOOD. I GRIEVED THAT MY WOMB THAT NEVER BORE CHILDREN AND NOW WITH MENOPAUSE THE LOSS OF ALL THAT POSSIBILITY. THE BLEEDING HAD ALWAYS SIGNIFIED SOME HOPE, AND I FELT AGAIN DEEP SADNESS, REGRET AND LOSS THAT I HAD NOT BORNE A CHILD. IT LEFT ME FEELING DEPLETE AS A WOMAN. THAT WAS THE FIRST DEATH. THE DEATH OF THAT HOPE.'

Liza

Everyone in menopause has to face the loss of their fertility, a real biological loss for sure, but tempered with different cultural meaning for each of us. Even with children, the sadness at this being the end of fertility can be haunting.

'I DO FEEL SAD ABOUT ONLY HAVING ONE CHILD. I PAY £300 A YEAR TO KEEP MY EMBRYOS FROZEN, KNOWING IT'S TOO LATE TO USE THEM.'

'Angie'

There are as many reasons for not having children as there are flowers in my garden and though the experience of child-loss and consciously choosing to be child-free are worlds apart, they share a similarity. Where most people are probably just interested and kind, the child-free can find themselves invaded by intrusive questions often coming from a defensiveness about the inquisitors' life choices.

'I CAN NOW LEGITIMATELY SAY TO PEOPLE, "IT'S TOO LATE FOR ME TO HAVE KIDS NOW", WHICH SHUTS THEM UP MORE EFFECTIVELY THAN SAYING, "I DIDN'T WANT TO HAVE CHILDREN." THANKS BIOLOGY!'

Emma

My hunch is that while fertility and motherhood are still perceived as a woman's primary means of creativity and meaning in life, there may not be much space for the grief of having lost children through miscarriage or not having been able to conceive a baby. All too often this sadness can become overwhelming through menopause, and an important part of the process is to give space for the grief to be expressed and acknowledged.

If you *have* had children, this too will affect your experience and it may not be the 'conventional' menopause layering of grief at having an empty nest. As more of us delay having children, or start second families in our mid-thirties, increasing numbers of us are dealing with toddlers while in perimenopause. Just when we need to retreat, it becomes impossible even to go to the loo without small attendants. This is a hard path.

I had what was charmingly known as a 'geriatric pregnancy', two of them in fact. There was the *Daily Mail* nipping at my heels, reminding me I'd left it too late. I was 40 at the time of the second birth and still recovering from the first, feeling traumatized and betrayed by my body and the system. With no family around and no contemporaries having had children at the same time as us, my partner and I struggled. Not having been much around babies meant I also didn't have any positive, empowering mothering role models. I struggled to find a way to be me and also a mother. I felt so lost. Like thousands of other new mums, swamped by the tide of small peoples' needs, oozing body fluid (mine and theirs), and pureed carrot, I longed for my urban professional self and my inner world to return. At which point the call to Separation came. The heart-pull of mothering and holding and wiping that caring for children brings pulled strong against my desire to run for the hills. I gazed with longing at ads for studio apartments, huts by the sea, and mountain retreats. As my cycle became more deeply Autumnal, I craved time out. I was securely enough attached to my partner and my children to hold this tension within myself. Feeling the pull, watching the thoughts and fantasies of going away, and feeling the love and bonds of care to hold these new little people as they grew.

How much support you had in your postnatal recovery and parenting *directly* influences your menopause experience. Being forced to get up, run around, and go back to work immediately after having your baby makes your symptoms worse and will affect your Second Spring vitality.

'MY CURRENT POSTMENOPAUSAL VITALITY IS 90 PER CENT BECAUSE I DIDN'T HAVE KIDS. IT'S SO HARD LOOKING AFTER ANOTHER HUMAN FOR TWENTY-FIVE YEARS. YOU'RE GIVING AWAY PART OF YOUR ESSENCE BY DELIVERING ANOTHER HUMAN BEING THROUGH THE PORTAL OF YOUR BODY, AND THAT'S GOING TO TAKE SOMETHING FROM YOU. WE DON'T GIVE THAT BACK TO WOMEN. IN CULTURES WHERE MOTHERS LIE IN AND ARE TAKEN CARE OF IN THE MONTHS AFTER THE BIRTH, THEY ARE BROUGHT BACK TO OPTIMAL HEALTH.'

Bryn Truett-Chavez, menopause mentor and cheerleader

In my observation of people in Second Spring, once biological fertility has ended and been processed emotionally, another wave of fertility naturally arises in the new cycle. Postmenopausal folk are richly fertile with new possibilities for their creativity; they take up pottery, start PHDs, climb mountains, and go cold water swimming. They create community projects, paint six-foot yonis, and sing in choirs – often all at the same time. It is simply untrue that all fertility ends at menopause; only that there will be no human babies coming out of there.

Practice

- Take time to reflect on a prompt that feels alive for you:
  - What does fertility mean to me?
  - What does the end of fertility mean to me?
  - What do I need to grieve?
  - What can I celebrate about my fertility?
  - You are fully entitled to employ your powers of discernment and to tell intrusive and judgemental people to get lost. You have nothing to apologize for or explain.
  - Connect with other people in the same situation; there's a Facebook group for everything.
  - Use the Self-Care Abdominal Massage (see pages 74–76) to connect with your womb space as a container for your creativity.

What might your body be asking of you?

39 Rage and grief

'MY SYSTEM WOULD BYPASS ALL THE
NORMAL LEVELS OF 'BEING' AND
GO STRAIGHT TO RAGE. RAGE STILL
SCARES ME IN OTHER PEOPLE, BUT
NOT IN MYSELF. IT'S A FEELING. MY
HEARTBEAT GOES CRAZY, I CAN FEEL
MY HEAD THROBBING AND I FEEL
OVERWHELMED WITH ANGER. I DON'T
PHYSICALLY HAVE TO DO ANYTHING
ABOUT IT. I SIT WITH IT, TRY AND
GET RID OF WHATEVER IS CAUSING
IT, BREATHE, AND WHEN IT'S
READY, IT LEAVES.'

Sharon

It's no surprise that the parody of menopause is a raging woman. You *will* be angry. Angry about dishwasher stacking and online forms, dog hair, climate change, and often without any particular cause at all. This is part of the Autumnal picture, just like the rages you may experience in your premenstrual Autumn. But what if we entertained the idea that our rage was justified? If we took these issues seriously and validated our feelings? Yes, it can feel overwhelming at times – because it's not just a few years of wet towels on the floor, it is *decades* of wet towels we're feeling.

'I'VE NOTICED I'M MUCH LESS FULL OF RAGE SINCE I'VE BECOME SINGLE. WHILST IN PERI AND MARRIED, RAGE WOULD RISE IN ME AND BE UNCONTROLLABLE. IT WOULD BE CYCLICAL, AND I WOULD USUALLY KNOW IT WAS COMING WHEN I NOTICED HOW UNTIDY THE HOUSE WAS. ABOUT ONCE A MONTH I WOULD HAVE THE NEED TO PURGE THE HOUSE OF CLUTTER OR RUBBISH, AND IF I COULDN'T OR IF SOMEONE CAME AND MESSED UP WHAT I HAD DONE OR JUST WEREN'T BEING HELPFUL, I WOULD GO INTO A COMPLETE MELTDOWN. THIS WOULD OFTEN CARRY THROUGH TO OTHER THINGS AND I WOULD SOMETIMES PICK A FIGHT WITH MY HUSBAND OR JUST EXPLODE WITH FRUSTRATION WHENEVER I FELT LET DOWN BY HIM OR HIS ACTIONS.'

Sandra

Perhaps because of cultural stereotypes, we are often afraid of our anger, fearing that if we let the lid off it, the force will be overwhelmingly destructive and uncontainable, to let loose all the firepower one has.

Menopause graciously teaches us to accept that our anger is valid and needs to be expressed, though it's not always skilful or tidy. Menopause is holding us in a process where she offers us tough love in the form of integrating our darker sides. You will have come across Second Spring folk who haven't made friends with their anger, whose tightly held bitterness simmers just below the surface, leaking out at the slightest scratch. This person will be having fewer warm Spring breezes and more of a miserable late frost because they are so busy keeping everything strapped down and under control.

'THE WILD WOMAN, WHO HAD ALWAYS BEEN WITH ME, WAS COMING THROUGH FAST AND FURIOUS. IT WAS ABOUT ME REALLY SAYING WHAT I WANTED, TAKING SELF-RESPONSIBILITY FOR HOW THINGS SHOULD GO.'

Sarah

Now that the oestrogenic veil has lifted, maybe it's not the towels that are the source of the rage; maybe it is the bigger picture. There will be worthy and righteous rage about the lack of value we hold for mothering, for our cyclical nature, for the desecration of the earth, for the pitiful way gender and sexuality are restricted, for the imbalance in wages, for structural racism, for the ravages of capitalism, or the awful, awful destruction of First Nation peoples. What has been manageable to hold on to during the Summer years of life can erupt volcanically in the Autumn and Winter. Clients often speak of feeling possessed, as though they have been taken over by the feelings and behaviour of another person.

Repressing our anger, which contains not only our natural expression but also the power to transform, can lead to depression. I have worked with many women who report feeling numb, depressed, or dead inside until they are able to access their rage. Perhaps it's no surprise that more than half of menopausal women report low moods and there are higher levels of depression in midlife. Think of the accumulation of fifty years' worth of repressed anger held inside a body. That takes a lot of energy to muffle, adding an extra burden of exhaustion at a sensitive time.

'OVER THE LAST FEW YEARS, I HAVE BECOME ALMOST VIOLENT IN MY HATRED OF THE WAY CHRISTMAS PERMEATES EVERYTHING FROM SEPTEMBER TO FUCKING FEBRUARY. IT'S ONE THING I CANNOT SIMPLY CHOOSE TO IGNORE BECAUSE EVERY FUCKER WANTS TO KNOW IF I'M READY FOR CHRISTMAS, WHAT MY PLANS ARE, WHY AM I NOT LOOKING FORWARD TO IT, AND WHETHER I HAD A LOVELY CHRISTMAS AND NEW YEAR (THIS LAST QUESTION IS ASKED WAY BEYOND THE POINT OF WHAT IS REASONABLE OR DECENT, IF YOU ASK ME).'

Emma

Following the shedding of masks, we have already seen how Autumn is the natural home for grief in the cycle. Separation will bring it in bucketloads. Loss of dewy skin, of opportunities and relationships, through miscarriages or abortions, of roads not travelled or years of illness, distraction or being trapped. Unfortunately, our culture is grief-averse. In the face of loss there's a push for us to buck up quickly, get over it and see the positive side. But the way through is by feeling it, by experiencing the feelings of loss one step at a time.

Another grief we encounter, especially if we've been lucky enough to be cycle aware, is the loss of our ovulation, our Inner Summer. That Wonder Woman week when nothing is too much and we're hot for sex *and* tidying. Will that ever return? Is it even reasonable to expect it to? At ovulation, for sure, we are more likely to feel that we are enough from the inside and also receive approval from the outside; one study showed that lap dancers earned a solid 81 per cent more in tips during ovulation than during their menstruation.[1] However, are we going to do sexy without it?

Clare Dubois, inspirational leader of Tree Sisters, is a great example, and kindly allowed me to use her words here:

Redefining 'She'

Wild One
I need you
Ready to shed your fear and thrive,
Ready to feel incandescently alive
Uncensored majesty of womankind
Embodying the grace of the sensually sublime
Receiver of nature's subtle melodies
Vivid, ageless, honest and free
I stand for you, and you stand for me
The redefined expression
Of appropriate 'She'.

Clare Dubois, founder of treesisters.org[2]

Practice

- Give yourself permission to grieve. Remember it is not a linear process and will come and go.
- Get help from friends, from family, and from professionals. It's important that your struggle is recognized and named.
- Jump over to chapter 45 and check out Tara Brach's RAIN Meditation.
- It helps if we can find safe ways to express our rage. In a 'formal' exercise class, you might imagine boxing and jumping on the imagined face of the 'evil one', aka the person who your rage is directed at. At home, you can try wringing out towels and biting into them, screaming and growling and moving in any damn way that feels good. If it doesn't feel safe to do it alone and you need more containment, there are loads of great facilitators and therapists who can hold a safe space for you to do this, have a look at the therapists in the Resources section. Expressing yourself through craft and art works well for some of us, or by writing poems or stories.
- Hot flushes can also be connected to anger. You may notice that your heat begins to rise in response to particular thoughts or situations. Can you use the heat of the flushing as an opportunity to experience the rage burning through you, out and away?

I have the right to feel and express whatever emotion I want.

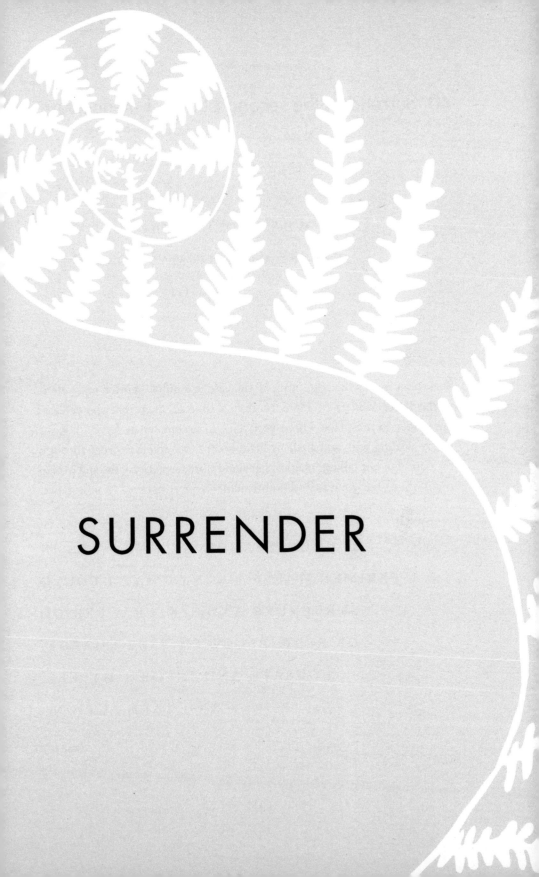

SURRENDER

40 Surrender: the second phase of menopause

'WHAT DOES SURRENDER FEEL
LIKE? GLORIOUSLY, NO LONGER
GIVING A FUCK!'

'Rachel'

Surrender marks the beginning of the Life Season of Winter, equivalent to the Inner Winter of menstruation, a time of deep rest and release. Surrender is the place where you start to accept whatever challenges you're dealing with and, little by little, acceptance starts to creep through the door. I'm not talking magical fairyland transformations, the shit-storm is still there, but your attitude subtly shifts from resistance to acceptance.

'UNDERSTANDING THAT I WAS IN
PERIMENOPAUSE MEANT THAT I COULD
SURRENDER AND, AFTER A PERIOD
OF REST, BEGIN TO TAKE CHARGE,
EDUCATE AND INFORM MYSELF,
AND TAKE ACTION.'

Jessica

Years ago, a very annoying therapist told me that resisting was harder work than letting go. It still irritates me twenty years later, but he was right in the sense that it *is* exhausting to resist change. Unfortunately, that doesn't exactly make it easier to enter Surrender. The sort of change you'll see is that instead of ignoring the 'problem', you start to ask, 'What do I need here?' You start to engage with the challenges that are knocking on your door, invite them in and give them a cup of tea, just like in the poem 'The Guest House' by the Sufi poet Jalaluddin Rumi:

This being human is a guest house.
Every morning a new arrival.

A joy, a depression, a meanness,
some momentary awareness comes
as an unexpected visitor.

Welcome and entertain them all! [1]

It's our relationship to the challenges that changes. Perhaps instead of pushing yourself to complete your massive to-do list, you start delegating or be more realistic about what you're able to achieve in a day. This is an ongoing experiment for me, in which I always hope to do more than I can and end up slightly disappointed in myself. My solution? I decide what is most important – meaning creative/fun/pleasurable – and do that first. If you're facing burnout or adrenal fatigue, perhaps you might start to consider the possibility of another career or going part time because your current way of working isn't sustainable.

Adrenal fatigue is common in menopause, the result of long-term stress or illness that leads to a fatigue that's not relieved by rest or sleep. It's not recognized by doctors until it becomes 'adrenal crisis' or Addison's disease, both of which can life-threatening. If you're wondering if adrenal fatigue is affecting you, have a look at the 'Self-help for hormones' table in chapter 3. Adrenal fatigue symptoms often swing between high and low cortisol, with a late-night high and morning low.

Whereas in Separation you try to rest and can't quite manage it, or not enough of it, in Surrender the quality and quantity of your rest improves. You find you are more committed to treating yourself kindly and can finally slow down and take deep rest.

'WITH ONE FOOT IN SEPARATION AND ONE IN SURRENDER, IT'S AN INTERESTING DANCE! IN SURRENDER THERE'S A TANGIBLE RELINQUISHING TO WHAT IS. WHEN I'M BACK IN SEPARATION, TENSION RISES IN MY BODY AND MY INNER CRITIC'S VOICE IS MUCH LOUDER. WHEN I SLIP OVER INTO SURRENDER, IT'S EASIER TO BE IN MY OWN HEADSPACE AND BODY, BE MORE ACCEPTING OF THE MANIFESTATIONS OF WHAT I NEED TO LET GO, AND OF THE EMOTIONS PASSING THROUGH. PROBABLY MOST IMPORTANTLY, I REST WITH MORE EASE IN SURRENDER.'

Leora Leboff

PRACTICE

- Use the Yoga Nidra for Surrender on pages 226–229.
- Use the Self-Care Abdominal Massage to invite softness and surrender to your belly (see pages 74–76).

Just. Let. Go.

Yoga Nidra for Surrender

This nidra will give you about 15 minutes of deep rest. Find a cosy space where you can recline undisturbed, with all the cushions and blankets you need, and as you read the practice through to yourself, let yourself be open as to what feels good for you. You might like to prop the book on a cushion, for example, so your arms and hands can relax.

GETTING READY

Welcome to the practice of yoga nidra.

Welcome to this safe, protected place of rest, your true home.

Just arriving here is enough, we've burned the to-do list and the hard part is over.

There is no wrong way to do this.

This is all just an invitation – if there's anything that doesn't sit well with you, you can let it go.

In this nidra you're going to get comfy, then explore the Seasons in the breath, check in with an inner smile; take a journey of feeling softness all around the body; explore pulsations of this softness; experience the inner journey of Surrender; check back in with an inner smile, the breath and then make your way back into the everyday world. All the time you'll be safe in your resting place.

GETTING COMFY

The intention of this practice is to accept the process of Surrender.

Hang up your 'do not disturb' sign, turn off your phone, and create a space to rest, gathering all the cushions and blankets you need to recline comfortably.

Wriggle around to find a position where your shoulders can release a bit more, softly settling back ...

Releasing the jaw with a yawn or a sigh.

Sinking into your resting place.

Letting your eyes soften.

Noticing the sounds beyond the place you are resting in.

Noticing the sounds in the space around you.

Drawing your attention closer to notice the sound of your breath.

THE SEASONS IN THE BREATH

Noticing the breath, the uniqueness of each breath, just soft and effortless ...

How each breath holds the Seasonal cycle, each one different and yet the same.

The start of the in-breath is the dawn of Spring;

Coming into the fullness of Summer;

Then releasing into the Autumn of the out-breath,

And the quiet of Winter at the end of the out-breath.

Notice how the Seasons roll effortlessly through the breath, the inevitability of it ...

The way your belly rises with the in-breath,

Always follows by the release and emptying of the out-breath;

Spring and Summer bringing you out into the world, and Autumn and Winter bringing you home to yourself ...

Name the Seasons of the breath for a few more cycles with the belly rising and falling.

Enjoy the Surrender as you breathe out ...

For a few breaths, bring your attention to the end of the out-breath,

Gently observing your breath as it comes and goes.

INNER SMILE

Take a moment to imagine that something good is coming your way, a pleasing sense of anticipation; good stuff is coming towards you ...

Notice how this feels in your body:

Like an inner smile.

KIND TOUCH AND REASSURANCE THROUGH THE BODY

Bringing your attention now to the body, we're going to take a journey, visiting places in the body and imagining they were each touched by a kind, reassuring touch.

A kind touch to the forehead between the eyebrows ...

To the jaw, the tongue and throat ...

Kind, reassuring touch for the right arm from the shoulder to each fingertip;

Kind, reassuring touch for the left arm from the shoulder to each fingertip;

A gentle touch for the torso, the collar bone, heart, navel, to the centre of the pubic bone;

Kind, reassuring touch for the right leg from the hip to the tip of each toe;

Kind, reassuring touch for the left leg from the hip to the tip of each toe.

Kindness pooling to fill the pelvic bowl ...

Then a reassuring touch to the base of the spine, the back of the waist, behind the heart, the top of the back, the shoulders –

The neck sweetly held;

And the gentlest of touches to each temple, each eye, the cheeks, nose and both sides of the jaw ...

The whole body is touched with a kind, reassuring touch.

PULSATIONS

On the in-breath, feel that the kindness expands to fill the whole body, and on the out-breath it draws back to fill the pelvic bowl.

Breathing in to expand the kindness all through;

Breathing out intensifies the kindness in the pelvis.

Moving between these two states,

The in-breath maybe expanding the kindness even beyond your body,

Each out-breath intensifying the kindness to the pelvic bowl.

Follow these pulsations for a few breath cycles …

Now holding both at the same time: both kindness expanding into the whole body and a deep, strong kindness centred in the womb. Both together. Noticing, for a moment, how it is to have both at the same time.

THE INNER JOURNEY OF SURRENDER

Imagine that you could journey down inside into the pelvic bowl, where you find you can rest in a safe, comfortable nest, with just the right kind of softness, just the right cushions and blankets for you to rest perfectly. Look how the gleaming, resilient structure of the pelvis encircles you and holds you safe, free from worries or cares. You are protected here. Take time to admire this beautiful home. Celebrating the resilience of a life lived, and survived. Finding in this safe citadel a place to rest, curling up now in this safe haven, you feel the protection of the pelvic bowl around you.

Deep inside this sacred space you find a golden seed, buried in layers of the sweetest aromatic wrappings, painted with intricate designs and symbols. This golden seed seems to pulsate with potency, yet is covered by a hard shell. The shell is intricate and beautiful and burnished, as though it has been polished and treasured over many years. You press the golden seed to your heart and in doing so it seems to vibrate and warm in your hands. It offers you the promise of a different way of being. Knowing you must take great care of this precious seed, you find the perfect place to plant it, deep, deep down back into the layers of aromatic wrappings. Each layered with blessings and gifts and resources to nourish her. Seeing her settling safe back down, resting in her beautiful shell until the Season for growth comes.

THE SEASONS IN THE BREATH

Noticing the breath once more …

How each breath holds the Seasonal cycle, each cycle different and yet the same:

The start of the in-breath the dawn of Spring,

Coming into the fullness of Summer,

Then releasing into the Autumn of the out-breath,

And the quiet of Winter.

Notice how the Seasons roll effortlessly through you, the inevitability of it,

The way your belly rises with the in-breath,

Always followed by the release and emptying of the out-breath.

INNER SMILE

Take another moment to imagine that something good is coming your way:

A warm openness ready to receive goodness.

Notice how this feels in your body:

Like an inner smile.

RETURNING TO THE HERE AND NOW

Noticing now the sound of your breath,

Expanding your attention to the sounds in the room around you ...

The sounds beyond the room as you come back into the here and now;

Start to expand your awareness of where you are, looking around at your space ...

Start to stretch and move, yawn and wriggle as you come back to the everyday world.

As we close this practice of yoga nidra, accept the process of Surrender.

Wide awake, wide awake and present.

Let yourself move gently from this yoga nidra, giving yourself space before you move back into your everyday life.

Congratulations on giving yourself this rest.

You will find a link for the audio for this nidra on p. 392.

41 Be with the Unknown

Have you ever found yourself worrying: 'What do I say when someone asks me what I've been doing?' It's a classic concern when we go against our culture of achievement by resting and giving our inner lives more attention. Our social interactions often highlight this conflict between the inner and outer worlds. The hoped for outcome is that your inner life is allowed more room, and that inner and outer ultimately can be better balanced in Second Spring. Perhaps the best answer to 'what have you been up to?' is 'a fabulous menopause transformation'.

The second aspect of Surrender is meeting the unknown. Having let go of our youth, goals, fertility, and maybe even our health, we see that our old ways of coping are definitely not working anymore, and we arrive in a new territory. We still don't know what will happen, which path to follow, or how to operate in the world, or who we will become. There is a brilliant courage in the acceptance of this Surrender; developing friendliness with the unknown will strengthen your spirit and set you free, because infinite possibilities can blossom from here. In the same way as you might go to the gym and focus on building upper-body strength, building the muscle of 'not knowing' brings you deeply into the experience of being alive. In truth, we are always on shaky ground, it's just that we choose to believe in the fantasy of control. For example, we might fantasize that if only we tried hard enough, we could be a size 10 again, or that if we could only eat enough broccoli we would never get ill. Spiritual seekers spend years reflecting on impermanence but in menopause, we're given the opportunity to put it into practice. Maybe the Tibetan Buddhist nun and acclaimed author Pema Chödrön was in menopause when she wrote:

To stay with that shakiness – to stay with a broken heart, with a rumbling stomach, with the feeling of hopelessness and wanting to get revenge – that is the path of true awakening. Sticking with that uncertainty, getting the knack of relaxing in the midst of chaos, learning not to panic – this is the spiritual path.[1]

'The path of true awakening' describes the phase of Surrender exactly, and of acknowledging that there is part of you who is totally cool with not knowing. Admittedly, this isn't always much help in the real world, where the pressures to decide what to do and to get over yourself are never far away.

The phases are never a linear process, however, and you'll find yourself flipping between Separation and Surrender on a daily, sometimes hourly, basis. To be in Separation after a week of Surrender is not a failure, though; it's being human. Separation is part of every cycle, and not something we can escape from, as much as we may long to be rid of it in menopause. It's the sign that something is getting ready to be released, a sign of change.

PRACTICE

Develop a friendship with the unknown by consciously connecting with your sense of not knowing.

- How does it show up in your body? If you feel numb, imagine what it might look like.
- Take a breath and get curious about it, feeling into how big it is, the texture and quality.
- Say hello to it.
- Greet it warmly and say, 'I see you, I love you', and notice what happens.
- Practice the Yoga Nidra for Surrender on pages 226–229.

Relax, everything is out of control.

42 Let go and listen

'LEARNING THAT PERI WAS SUPPOSED TO BE A BIT OF A MESS HELPED ME RELAX AND ACCEPT IT ALL, RATHER THAN FIGHT IT. THIS WAS HUGE.'

'Siobhan'

Surrender brings deep listening to our inner needs. How many times have you been told to 'listen to your body'? It sounds so simple, doesn't it: have a drink of water or a little nap, maybe? But it's much less easy to *really* follow through, because it's often inconvenient for other people. If you notice, for example, that doing the emotional labour in your relationship contributes to your fatigue, following through the necessary changes is hard work! There's negotiating, there's the fall-out from family, there's whinging and probably resentment. Your nearest and dearest, though they love you dearly, will seldom suggest that you let go of anticipating their needs and put your own needs first instead.

'I FINALLY REALIZED IT WAS TIME
FOR ME TO STEP UP AND BECOME
AN ADVOCATE FOR MYSELF.'

'Jo'

Deep listening and the action that follows require that we ground our-selves deep into something good within us, and we all do this differently. It might be your religious faith or perhaps a trust in your own goodness or the rhythm of the earth; however we individually feel it, through this reconnection with a central well of goodness and trust, we start to experience a stronger sense of being held by something bigger than us.

'TRUST HAS BEEN A BIG
COMPONENT OF MY JOURNEY.
TRUSTING LIFE, MYSELF, MY BODY.
AS A RECOVERING CONTROL PERSON,
THE ABILITY TO SURRENDER
INTO A DEEPER KNOWING THAT LIES
WITHIN AND LISTENING TO THAT
HAS ALLOWED ME TO UNFOLD MORE
INTO MY AUTHENTIC SELF.'

Nancy

If Separation is hearing that we need to care for ourselves, Surrender is actually listening and doing it. We know we should slow down and be mindful. Everybody knows that. Surrender happens when we *actually* slow down enough, usually way beyond what we think is reasonable; this is deep listening. It's an ongoing commitment to kindness in action instead of theory. The kindness of Separation is to go to bed a bit earlier; the kindness of Surrender is to go to bed for a weekend.

Surrender is a Wintery place, a place of dreaminess, rest, of dropping below into dreamy places – much like when you have, or used to have, your period.

'I WAS VERY LOW, I FELT NO ONE WOULD WANT ME, I WAS PAST IT. WHAT CHANGED THAT FOR ME WAS THAT I LAY DOWN AND UNDERSTOOD THAT IT WAS AN INITIATORY JOURNEY AND THEN EVERYTHING CHANGED; I KNEW I HAD TO LET GO OF WHO I THOUGHT I WAS.'

Edwina Staniforth, activist and herbalist

We have become too tired to pretend to be the person we think other people will love. For many people, it's their primary relationship where the letting go happens, realizing that they can't, after all, turn their partner into the person they wish they'd married. Or finding that masking their sexual preference or neurodiversity is just not worth the cost. Or that looking a particular way to please someone else is a waste of time, as are tiny things like the effort that can go into matching socks. Surrender is standing naked without the defences that have served us so well over the years. We arrive at trust by a hard route.

'STAY TRUE TO WHO YOU ARE
AND WHAT YOU REALLY WANT.
THERE IS NO OTHER WAY THROUGH
MENOPAUSE THAN THROUGH THIS
ROUTE; NO SHORT CUTS, ONLY DEEP
COMMITMENT TO WHO YOU ARE
MOMENT BY MOMENT.'

Alexandra Pope, co-founder of Red School

PRACTICE
- Use the Clearing Meditation on pages 54–56 to assist in your letting go.
- Use the Circle process (see chapter 16) to find out how you can listen and understand what is ripe for release in your life.
- Do your favourite yoga nidra.
- Give yourself a Self-Care Abdominal Massage (see pages 74–76). Use your hands to really listen to yourself, and feel the letting go beneath your hands.

Stand naked and proud; the time for shame is over.

43 Birth your self

You can't make yourself surrender. It doesn't work that way, just as you can't make yourself birth your baby at exactly forty weeks. But birthing yourself in Surrender has some lovely parallels to birthing a baby, which can be helpful to think about:

- You need to feel safe and able to absolutely trust the people around you.
- You need to find your own rhythm and pace, trusting your body to do the work.
- You need to be educated in the process; remember that you are in a Seasonal process of rebirth and even though it may look like nothing is happening in this time of Winter, you are in a fertile emptiness.
- You need calm; adrenalin from people around you will interrupt the process.
- Stay with the sensations; just as using the 'thinking mind', the neocortex, halts labour, staying with the sensations keeps you in the zone.
- Loving touch – stroking, massage and hugging – all support oxytocin flow in menopause process.
- Pleasure is key for supporting oxytocin flow in birth – and I'd put money on masturbation being key for menopause too.

- It needs to be quiet; shouty people demanding stuff from you will halt the process.
- Let go of your expectations. Then lower them some more.

Any takers for an orgasmic menopause? No, really! The dismissal of menopausal and postmenopausal women as non-sexual beings says more about cultural bias than real lived experience. Listening to my clients, they say their sexuality has changed and they are needing to learn new ways to pleasure themselves. To catch up with what their body needs. There's more on this in chapters 49 and 50, but pleasure and orgasm have body-wide benefits, such as strengthening your pelvic floor, reducing inflammation, increasing happy hormones such as serotonin, helping you sleep better, and boosting testosterone levels. If we're going to rewrite the meno-script, let's make it a good one!

PRACTICE
- Make yourself a 'do not disturb' sign to put on your door.
- Using the same requirements for birth, safety and quiet etc, explore how your body would like to be touched, what gives you pleasure right now?
- Use the Self-Care Abdominal Massage and touch yourself with all the love and tenderness you'd give to a pregnant woman.
- Write a letter to the person you would love to birth, welcoming them into the world.

I am giving birth to my new self.

44 Self-care for Surrender

'CARING FOR MYSELF IS NOT
SELF-INDULGENCE, IT IS SELF-
PRESERVATION AND THAT IS AN ACT
OF POLITICAL WARFARE.'

Audre Lorde, A Burst of Light[1]

Self-care looks different for everyone. Sometimes it can become a heavy burden on your must-do list or even a slightly toxic indulgence. We need to find the ways that feel truly kind for us, which includes sometimes saying *fuck it all* and ditching the whole business for a bag of crisps instead. Yes, crisps can be self-care too. Self-care is not about spending lots of money or about saving up for a day relaxing in a spa when you work like a dog the rest of your life. It's about care for your self, responding to your needs from a place of kindness and love, treating yourself as you would your best friend. It's all those small daily practices of gentleness that will support and nourish you through this sensitive time.

Generally speaking, your kind self-care will fall into these categories:

- A regular mindful practice such as mindfulness, yoga, being in nature, Self-Care Abdominal Massage, or breathwork etc.
- Nourishing movement – the kind of exercise that makes you happier.
- A good structure of health professionals, complementary and/or medical.

- Kind self-talk or at least a growing awareness of how the harmful self-talk operates within you.
- Let go of your expectations for yourself, then let go some more.
- Spending dedicated time looking inward – therapy, journaling, meditating, yoga, a listening partnership, dream diaries… There's a way for every pocket and taste.
- Find and do more of what soothes your soul.
- Say no to even more stuff – there are some subtle ways of saying no in chapter 59.

'DEEP, DARK, WITH THE REAL MESSY ME RIGHT AT THE BOTTOM, WAITING TO BE LET UP INTO THE LIGHT AGAIN. AS I REGULARLY DID MENOPAUSE MEDITATIONS, I CAME TO VALUE THE QUIET AND DARK FOR LISTENING IN AND HELPING ME FACE TRUTHS.'

Sarah

By now you will have become an expert in your unique blend of self-care. The only difference in Surrender is now it has become a given, not an option. You can see increasing chunks of time where you can drift, tend sweetly to your aches, let go of or screen out what disturbs you, and become better acquainted with not knowing what on earth is going on. Self-care equals kind words, self-compassion, soothing, and pleasure, whatever that means to you. Here's a checklist as a reminder:

- more space
- less stress
- kindness
- more pyjama time
- good company
- good food
- pleasure
- saying no
- drifting
- daydreaming
- slack-jawed gazing
- sleep – if you can get it
- resting more anyway
- clearing toxicity from your environment
- observing your distress with a kindly and wry eye
- moving in ways that please you
- clearing emotional toxicity

Bringing the kindness of Surrender to a weary menopausal traveller is a bit like hugging a child that's bumped its knee. In fact, it is exactly like that because you will be tending in an everyday way to your inner self. Each act of kindness towards yourself – saying no to things that exhaust you, enjoying a quiet cup of tea, a bit of sweet self-talk in the mirror – will soften your tension. Your shoulders will melt, your heart will open and the parts of you that hurt will be a little more soothed each time. It's as though your inner self starts to trust your everyday self more and more. That you really mean it this time. The combination of deep listening and familiarity with the unknown brings a sweet intimacy with yourself, so you can finally find peace and begin to trust that life and the Seasonal cycle have your back.

PRACTICE

- Use the Circle process (see chapter 16) to identify your personal prescription for Surrender.
- Use the Yoga Nidra for Surrender (see pages 226–229).
- Give yourself a Self-Care Abdominal Massage (see page 74), but do it even more slowly and with even more love than last time.

What might soothe you right now?

45 Heal those wounds

Surrendering gives us the opportunity to heal wounds that are just too impossible to think about addressing when we're in a Separation phase. Menopause is a magnet for unresolved issues in your life. We are bowled over by psychological changes and also by the unexpected accidents, arguments, fallings-out, triggers, and the general weirdness that shows up at this time. All kinds of events seem to cluster together now that we wouldn't necessarily associate with menopause. I've lost count of the times people said that they happened to move to a new area at this time, or their relationship ended, or they were bereaved. In the mainstream world such events are perceived as incidental, but as we understand that menopause is a psychological process of growth, we can see that our attitude to these issues are emerging from within us for resolution. It's not just because life's a bitch.

'IT'S LIKE A TAX RETURN, THE GREAT SELF-ASSESSMENT; FESS UP! PAY WHAT YOU OWE!'

Uma Dinsmore-Tuli, activist and author of Yoni Shakti

The solution is simple; your path is to feel the feelings. That's it. Unfortunately, humans have a *slight* tendency to move away from emotional pain because we think it's going to hurt us, possibly fatally. Like in Michael Rosen's story *We're Going on a Bear Hunt*, we have tricky terrain to cross, long grass, sticky mud – and each time finding we can't go under it, we have to go through it. This is how we need to meet our feelings to move towards healing.

Our emotions are like those scary subways under busy roads: you have to brave the darkness, the unknown, and the smell of wee to get to the light at the other end. Sometimes it's easier than we expect, sometimes it hurts like hell, and very often there is judgement arising about having our feelings at all. This is where practising non-judgement comes in, as we saw in chapter 33. But we do have a great ally, in that the absence of oestrogen can also give us more clarity about what belongs in the past and what needs dealing with now.

The women i work with who are experiencing difficult menopause, for some of them it is the first time that they have really listened to their bodies and there is so much held in them which needs to be expressed, released and transformed.

Suzanne Yates, founder of Wellmother

The issues pressing to be expressed are built into our physiology, in our brains – the amygdala and hippocampus are sensitive to hormonal fluctuations – which may be why old memories surface at this time of life.

Trauma

If you are a trauma survivor, entering into healing old wounds requires great respect and care, and you may choose to find professional help as you navigate the healing that menopause requires. Somatic Experiencing, also known as 'SE', is a therapy that focuses on the sensation in the body and offers an effective and gentle way of working with difficult emotions, as do mindfulness or a more cognitive approach such as CBT. CBT is a talking therapy that focuses on how your beliefs and thoughts can contribute or help with your issue. If you feel that you're feeling fairly steady, then Trauma Release Exercises can be helpful. These use a gentle shaking to release the muscle memory of the trauma and you can find a practitioner, a workshop or look it up on YouTube. Also known as TRE, the exercises can be beneficial for anyone to use to release tension and soothe the nervous system.

You are doing OK

Life can be hard; each and every one of us is wounded and knows pain. There's even a possibility that the more traumatic experiences you had as a child, the worse your menopause experience might be. In whatever ways that you approach your vulnerabilities you are doing OK – really,

really OK. Life can be hard work, menopause especially, so never let anyone tell you you're not doing your healing right, or enough, or with the correct method. You are doing OK just as you are and there is no need to add another layer of shame and wounding on top of what you're dealing with.

PRACTICE

- Journaling prompt: how are my old wounds showing up in my life now?
- Explore using the RAIN Meditation (see pages 246–247), or try TRE, and see if either or both approaches suit you. If you're not into them, explore other ways of encountering and releasing difficult feelings; there's a book list in the Resources section for inspiration.
- If you need professional help, see what you feel drawn to; perhaps you'd prefer a cognitive, body or mindfulness approach.
- Some prefer a self-directed way through, probably something that you already enjoy doing, like dancing or drawing.

Imagine if you just
accepted the way you
felt, and were OK with
it? Radical!

RAIN Meditation

Mindfulness teacher Tara Brach's RAIN Meditation is a wonderful way of encountering difficult feelings; she calls it an 'in-the-trenches support for working with intense and difficult emotions', which you can use wherever you need to become present to yourself and your feelings.[1] It's a four-step process:[2]

R – Recognize what is happening
A – Allow things to be just as they are
I – Investigate your inner experience with kindness
N – Nurture

Here's how it has worked for me when I was furiously shouty with my youngest child because she was prioritizing scrolling over clearing up the mess she'd left in the kitchen ...

Recognize: I paused to check out what was happening inside me and noticed how I had a tight, hot feeling in my diaphragm and belly. Trying not to judge, I got interested in the precise shape and texture of this tightness.

Allow: the allow part is pretty radical. It asks us to accept what is happening as it is; in this case, it was my rage, my daughter's hurtful words, my feelings of being a crap parent ... just letting it all be there and saying 'yes' to it. You will want to find your own words: 'Oh yes, this is how it is', or something else. I resonate with 'I see you'.

Investigate: next, I gave some time to feel into the texture of the tightness, where it began and ended, what happened as I breathed into it. An alternative might be to ask, 'What needs to happen here?' or 'How can I bring kindness to the situation?' and see what arises. The trick is to avoid getting caught up in the story or in blame, but to investigate your feelings kindly as you might a toddler with a bumped head. I realized that my daughter and I had got too much in each other's faces; we needed more space.

Nurture: as a result of the RAIN meditation I was able to feel tender towards both myself and my girl, and to understand how we both needed space – she to find ways to grow into the adult she's becoming, and me to move away from my role as mother. This acknowledgement and space were nurturing and I gave myself some kind self-talk too.

You can find Tara Brach doing a 10-minute RAIN Meditation on her site.[3] After a few practices, you will be able to use the RAIN Meditation any time you feel you're in need of solace.

One of the advantages of RAIN is that it enables us to manage difficult feelings when it's necessary to hold everything together. Even when we're on a focused self-healing mission, we don't necessarily want to dive deep into our material at the cost of getting the kids to school or showing up for work. Using RAIN, we can dilute our feelings more manageably.

Let body intelligence lead the way.

46 Small kindnesses make for big change

'I DON'T THINK YOU CAN DEAL WITH OTHER
PEOPLE'S PROBLEMS UNTIL YOU HAVE PUT ON
YOUR OWN OXYGEN MASK. SELF-CARE AND
SELF-KINDNESS ARE ESSENTIAL AND SHOULD
BE PRACTISED ON A DAILY BASIS.'

'Lucy'

Humans are like Velcro for negative thinking and Teflon for positive thinking: somehow the bad stuff just seems stickier. This means we have to put extra effort into working our self-kindness muscle. One of the most powerful ways we use for growing kindness at Woman Kind is to ask our participants to commit to one small kindness that they can do every day.

I HAVE NO WISH TO BE PART OF THINGS
OR PEOPLE THAT ARE NOT ALIGNED
WITH WHERE I'M AT. I'VE BECOME LESS
BOTHERED BY WHAT OTHERS REQUIRE
FROM ME AND MY FUCK-IT MONITOR
SEEMS TO BE CONSTANTLY ON.

'Kate'

We learned this from our training at menstrual educators Red School, where it's known as the 1 per cent. So, if what you really long for is to live in the Caribbean, your 1 per cent might be spending a little time outside in nature every day or buying yourself some flowers at the supermarket. It might be a walk outside, taking a conscious breath, or doing a yoga stretch before bed; any small, doable thing.

Then we just sit back and watch the magic happen, because from that one doable act of kindness, we take baby steps towards more – and before long we observe massive leaps forwards in consciousness; the 'homeopathic' daily micro dose works its magic. For example, one woman who decided to smile at herself in the mirror instead of giving herself negative talk has eventually come to feel comfortable in her body for the first time in her life.

Research into building new habits confirms that the best way to create change is to make specific, tiny, doable steps and to integrate them into something you already do. Having your commitment to yourself witnessed by non-judgemental friends also supports you in following through.

'SELF-KINDNESS, FOR ME, IS ACCEPTING MYSELF AS I AM AND NOT STRIVING FOR A NON-ATTAINABLE PERFECTION. IT INVOLVES TAKING MY OWN NEEDS AS SERIOUSLY, EVEN MORE SERIOUSLY, THAN ANYONE ELSE'S. PRACTICALLY, THIS INVOLVES ENSURING I GET ENOUGH SPACE AND TIME FOR MY PROCESSES, EATING NOURISHING FOOD, SEEKING THE COMPANY OF GOOD AND KIND FRIENDS, AND SPENDING MY TIME IN ACTIVITIES I LOVE — BEING IN NATURE, WALKING WITH MY DOG, YOGA, TAI CHI, AND READING.'

'Alison'

Two words of warning, though. When you commit to your small kindnesses, it's easy to beat yourself up when you forget. Try to catch self-criticism before it runs away with itself, and remind yourself that if someone had taught you self-kindness to begin with, then you'd know how to do it already. You're only human after all. Another thing that can happen is that by committing to the kindness, its opposite manifests; for example, when learning to adore your appearance, you might encounter criticism about the way you look from a family member. This is healing in action: your issues arising to reveal to you how they operate. If this happens, pay close attention and observe how the dynamic unfolds … and keep on being kind to yourself.

PRACTICE

- Breathe all the way out now, and as you breathe in, place one hand on your heart and one on your lower belly. After a few soft breaths, ask yourself, 'What kindness can I give myself?' and see what emerges. When you have settled on a small, specific, doable kindness, write it down on a Post-it Note where you'll see it, make it your screen saver, or share it with a friend.
- When you're inspired to journal, try writing on this topic: 'It's hard to be kind to myself because ...'

Small changes are proven to be a more sustainable way to create change.

47 Your menopausal partner needs you

The effect of menopause transition ripples out towards our nearest and dearest, and our partners are strongly affected too. Practically everyone I've met in menopause has struggled in their relationship as wounds come up for healing. While we feel adrift from ourselves and struggle to cope with strong feelings, our partners can feel abandoned in our slipstream as we feel Separation calling us away. Hopefully, they are just longing to know how they could help us, but if we can't communicate skilfully because screaming the truth is the only way we can do it now (ouch!), then it can be really hard to weather the storm together.

Couples therapist and trainer Joanna Groves talks about finding a common language that you can use to describe your experience, which dips beneath the regular blaming that can get in the way and which can bring your partner on board as an ally instead – more 'I need more time to myself' than 'pair your own bloody socks'. The alienation that our partners can feel happens regardless of gender, or even regardless of whether they themselves have experienced menopause; it's just that a person in the menopause process is necessarily withdrawing into themselves, because that is part of the process.

On your behalf, when you need your partner to be an ally, you can show them this letter:

Dear partner to a menopausal person,

You probably feel that you've lost the person you fell in love with, that she's drifted away from you, and changed beyond recognition. Please do not despair – she will come back even more beautiful than before, in her own time. Like the caterpillar, she has to build herself a cocoon to withdraw into, where she can dissolve and then re-form herself into a butterfly.

For quite a while, she is going to be mush inside the cocoon and not ready to come out: poking her won't do it; asking her to do all the 'looking after' tasks she used to do won't do it; suggesting antidepressants won't do it; and trying to fix her won't do it. What she needs is for you to act as her cocoon, to help her create strong boundaries and to hold her while she changes and works out who she's going to be. This might mean you have to take on some of the tasks she used to do, giving her more space, more peace and, most of all, giving her time. Your partner needs you now more than ever, even though she probably can't express this skilfully to you.

Part of the mushy period is about healing old wounds and trauma, so problems will probably show up in your relationship. Trust that these new challenges have arisen so they can be healed for both of you; your capacity to be open to hearing how she feels is pure gold to her and will take your relationship to deeper levels of intimacy.

You may find yourself scared by the changes you see in her; she's looking at what is working and what is not working in her life. This process will help her to become more of herself, to be both powerful and vulnerable, playful and a player, to expand into aspects of her being that have been ignored or shamed before. As well as holding the space, your task is to do the same. Identify what is nourishing for you and to move towards what your soul longs for. She is stepping up her game and to have a meaningful relationship, you must step up yours too. Here are some wise words from Nico, a perimenopausal woman:

The main thing is, take your partner seriously and don't blame all her moods and feelings on her hormones. There is more to menopausal women than hormonal changes and many of them have a good reason to be very angry, tired, and confused. Please step up and help more with childcare, elderly care, etc. Honour and respect this woman who works so hard in all of the ways, and never say, 'Oh, it's just her hormones.'

Menopause takes a little time, but if you can stay steady, she will return to you twice the woman she used to be, radiant with life.

PRACTICE

Here are some of the things that might help your menopausal partner:

- Leave dark chocolate near her and run away.
- Take over as many of the domestic tasks as you can.
- Give her space and quiet, and trust that she will return to you in time.
- Listen to how she feels without trying to fix her.
- Tell her she's doing great.

She will come back to you in her own time, even more beautiful than before.

48 Sex can get worse

One of oestrogen's lovely qualities is to make our tissues plump and juicy. As our oestrogen levels decline, our skin becomes dryer, more fragile, and we have less collagen to play with. It's true of our faces and also true of our vulvas and vaginas. The grim term 'vaginal atrophy', brilliantly reframed by clinical hypnotherapist Sophie Fletcher as having a 'trophy vagina',[1] describes a condition with a spectrum from dryness through to constant pain that can make sitting or even wearing clothes unbearable; but 50 per cent of menopausal women experience it at some time and it can start early in perimenopause.[2] Like the vagina herself, a lot of this stays hidden; because of its intimate nature, few women feel able to approach their doctors to talk about it.

'I DON'T THINK I REALLY DROPPED FULLY INTO MY CALLING UNTIL I REACHED MENOPAUSE AND I FOUND OUT THAT I WAS EXPERIENCING VULVOVAGINAL ATROPHY; THERE HAD BEEN CONSIDERABLE "LOSS" TO THE OUTER LABIA. THE PAINFUL SEX PREVIOUS TO THIS EVENT TURNED OUT TO BE A TELL-TALE SIGN. MY OWN EXPERIENCES BROUGHT ME TO MY CALLING AND I'M ETERNALLY GRATEFUL THAT 'SHE' HAS SHOWN THE WAY AND GIFTED ME HER WISDOM, LOVE, AND GENEROSITY.'

Andrea Clarke, Holistic Pelvic Care® therapist

There's a variety of symptoms that include labia shrinking or disappearing, urinary tract infections, burning sensations, vaginal dryness, painful sex, itching, splitting skin, and unpleasant discharge. Many women suffer greatly from incorrect diagnosis and treatment. One interviewee, Karen, said:

> *I feel like my vagina is speaking loudly; she says NO! I do not want to have a penis or anything else inside me unless there is a deep intimacy established first. Before perimenopause my body used to comply, but not anymore.*

Our poster girl for vaginal atrophy is Jane Lewis, whose book *Me and My Menopausal Vagina* is full of useful information and ideas about how to manage the condition.[3] If you suffer from this debilitating condition, read it. If you don't suffer from it, read it; it will give you a deep gratitude for your amazing vulva and nurture understanding for the other half of the vulva owners who experience this condition. Jane also has an excellent support group on Facebook.

Our bodies talk and that talk becomes louder as we age, speaking of what happens when we keep ourselves small and carry the shame of generations of women. Could it be that the historical shaming of women's sexuality is being played out in the 50 per cent of the female population who suffer from vaginal atrophy? We'll never know, of course. But my bright vision of the future is that the shame is lifted and we are free to express our sexuality in any way we wish; while at menopause, our vaginas and vulvas are concerned only with pleasure. While we're waiting for this situation to manifest, because it might take a generation or so, testosterone cream can work wonders for the libido, with few side effects.

'OVERNIGHT I CHANGED
FROM A SEXUALLY EXPRESSIVE
PERSON, IT FELT LIKE SOMEONE
HAD TURNED THE SWITCH OFF. IT
WAS HEART-BREAKING AND PUT ME
INTO A STATE OF GRIEVING.'

Lillian

Topical oestrogen works very well for many women with vaginal atrophy and holds none of the risks associated with HRT as it's very low dose. 'Clara', an interviewee who had been suffering with tears in her vaginal wall, reported after using it:

'I feel like I've got a brand-new vagina!'

If you prefer not to use topical oestrogen, lubes or moisturisers can be enough if your symptoms are not severe. The takeaway from Jane Lewis is that there's no one-size-fits-all solution and that there are many different things to try if you wish to find out what works for you.

PRACTICE

- Journaling prompt: what does your vagina want to say? What's she pissed off about? What does she long for?
- Don't let any kind of soap or scented product near your vulva, as these act as irritants.
- Keep your whole pelvis area vital and full of energy: consulting with a women's health physiotherapist, and/or

practising women's yoga, Holistic Pelvic Care® (a bodywork practice created by Tami Lynn Kent), belly dancing, any dancing, Hypopressives (special core exercises) or abdominal massage are all great for this.

- Exercise wisely and practise a form of meditation.
- Introduce the following sources of supportive nutrients into your diet: fenugreek sprouts, linseeds, sesame seeds, and sea buckthorn capsules, along with Vitamin E.

Don't suffer in silence: let your vagina speak her truth.

49 Sex can get much, much better

Let's bust another myth – that after menopause all women go off sex. Wrong. Knackered women go off sex. Stressed women go off sex, as do women in relationships that have grown stale, or where abuse has surfaced for healing; in relationships with unresolved issues, where women are or have been shamed, been told they are ugly or body shamed, or have body dysmorphia. It is not the menopause putting us off sex: it's a time of transformation when we simply cannot go on as we have before.

As we reach menopause we will not put up with lazy attempts at foreplay – we need to be seen, to be met with heart and mind, and only then maybe with genitals too. Many women I interviewed reported that they were having the best sex of their lives at menopause and beyond, because they now have the wisdom to understand what suits them and the authority to ask for it. Having said that, it's worth pointing out that that none of them were in long-term relationships.

'IN PERIMENOPAUSE I HAD A RESURGENCE OF SEXUAL ENERGY. IT WAS WONDERFUL AND VERY LIBERATING. I LITERALLY FELT KUNDALINI ENERGY RISING IN ME DURING A MEDITATION ONE DAY. I REMEMBER BECAUSE I WAS WITH FRIENDS AND WE WERE TRYING TO WORK OUT WHAT IT WAS! IT WAS A VERY NEW EXPERIENCE AND MOST WELCOME. DEFINITELY THE BEST THING TO COME OUT OF PERI.'

Sandra

Another myth that obscures our real, lived experience of sexuality in menopause is that expressing our libido only equates with encountering a penis in vagina sex. No. Our libido is our life force and includes our creativity, our ideas, the way we love our friends, our words, and our capacity for sensual pleasure of all kinds. If you look around you, you'll notice that those in Second Spring are having a lot of fun.[1] If we think of sexual energy in the broadest possible context, depending on your belief system you might call it 'life force' as I do, or 'Source energy', chi or prana; it then becomes easy to see that the health and vitality of our sexuality is utterly bound up with the health and vitality of our lives. In other words, if you want good sex, start with what makes you feel alive and the fun will follow.

'I FEEL LIKE ALL MY SEXUAL ENERGY IS NEEDED FOR MY PERSONAL CREATIVITY, AND I'M BEING QUITE SELFISH ABOUT THIS.'

Jessica

If your libido has dropped away, you may have to take time to get reacquainted with what is pleasurable for you now, and this requires time, safety, lube – and no agendas. You could take yourself on a date, enjoy candles, savour your favourite food, wear your favourite underwear, and get curious and explore your body. Masturbation is self-care with so many benefits; it brings circulation to the vulva and vagina to help maintain tone, releases endorphins (our natural painkillers), reduces stress (which will help rebalance your endocrine system), helps you sleep, improves your mental health, and much more. You can use your hands, or a toy, or wand, or anything you like – as long as it feels good for you in the moment.

It is true that lower oestrogen levels thin the labia and inside of the vagina, but once you're armed with lube, this just means that your sexual needs have changed, not that they've disappeared. It's the start of a whole new sexual adventure, discovering for ourselves what feels good now, as the person we are now, or are becoming.

The spectrum of 'normal' is super wide, and at one end the libido can skyrocket with pleasure running the show. Think of artist Molly Parkin, in her eighties, sharing that she started each day with an orgasm before she got back to her painting in her studio.[2,3] In *The Menopause Monologues 2*, Lucy recalls:

> *At the gym I'd have to use the cross-trainer next to the window to avoid drooling over the toned hunks working out beside me. I went to the gym a lot. I discovered that a hard workout was just about the only way to achieve temporary respite from my raging hormones.*[4]

At other end of the spectrum, it's a relief not to be 'driven' by sexual needs anymore. Like Gloria Steinem said, it leaves your mind 'free for all kinds of things'.[5]

'I HAVE SO MANY MORE INTERESTING PROJECTS TO GIVE MY ENERGY TO, I'M AMAZED I USED TO WASTE SO MUCH TIME AND ENERGY PURSUING SEX.'

'Sally-Ann'

Wherever you are, you are OK.

PRACTICE

- Use lube to explore by yourself and/or with your partner. See the Resources section for some great organic buys.
- Explore what messages you have absorbed about your body and your sexuality from your family and culture. How has this impacted your feelings about your sexuality? What aspects would you like to let go of?
- How do you long for your sexuality to be expressed?
- Use the Self-Care Abdominal Massage on pages 74–76 as often as you can to reconnect with pleasurable touch.
- Holistic Pelvic Care® or abdominal massage sessions can help to heal sexual wounds and trauma; you will find details in the Resources section.

Take time to pleasure yourself.

50 Contraception

If you are in a sexual relationship with a man and don't want to have a baby, you're going to need a plan. It's not uncommon for the unpredictability of perimenopause to allow for some surprise babies; Cherie Blair popped one out in Downing Street, for example, while Tony Blair was prime minister, much to the tabloids' delight. As soon as you heard the news, you couldn't not imagine them having sex. Similarly, a friend told me the story of how her mum became pregnant in 1960s Liverpool when she thought she was in menopause in her forties, and the parish priest came to the house and told her she was a disgrace for still having sex at that age. Though she wasn't a churchgoer, she sent her kids to the local Catholic school and it turned out that the nuns there had reported her to the priest.

As I started to research this topic, I found, yet again, that contraception in perimenopause was just not talked about. All the research seems to be done into the effects on younger women – no surprise there. I started to wonder if the old story of sexual shame was still running along underground. Contraception, never an easy or straightforward choice, becomes even trickier as the fertile years draw to a close.

The medical advice seems straightforward: to be absolutely sure there are no surprise buns in your oven, you'll need to use contraception for at least two years after your last period if you're under 50. If you are lucky enough to be over 50, then use contraception for one year following your last period. If you're not menstruating after 55, it's a free-for-all sex-fest and no contraception is required. HRT is not a contraceptive unless it's the kind where you're not having periods; in which case you are unlikely to need contraception, but check with your doctor regarding your particular situation.

So far so linear. But our cycles are not simply physiological events: they are also invitations to get intimate with ourselves and to heal, and as such, are seldom regular or predictable. Periods can stop and start and stop again, sometimes with long gaps between them, especially during perimenopause. Ovulation comes and goes too, and even after many cycles without an egg popping, you can be surprised by your ovaries squeezing another one out.

Talking about contraception, it seemed that choices were often blown off-course by our internal, emotional conflicts. For example, the grief for our departing fertility often gets played out as 'carelessness' in not using contraceptives consistently. If you have left a long-term relationship and are exploring new sexual adventures, all sorts of issues can arise, evidenced by the increasing number of abortions in the 40+ age bracket, despite the need to protect ourselves from sexually transmitted diseases.[1,] [2] According to menopause advocate Meg Mathews, in the States, it's common to have the results of your sexual health exam accessible on your phone[3] so that you and your partner can check each other out and be sure of being safe[4], but I've not yet encountered this straightforward approach in the UK.

When the pill was first available, it was heralded as liberation. Which it was, up to a point. Maybe in the same sense that a brick through a prison window might let in a refreshing breeze. There's now a huge range of contraception to choose from, something for everybody. As long as they're used correctly you can be up to 99 per cent sure you won't get pregnant, but there can be hidden side effects and issues that come with hormonal contraception.

First off, if you are taking hormonal contraception, you won't have much of an idea if you're in menopause or not, or what menopause phase you might be in. The effect of taking artificial hormones will be to make the Seasonal swing of both your menstrual and your Life Seasons less obvious to you. If your experience of the menstrual Seasons is super challenging and your life is already too much, then hormonal contraception can be a brilliant choice, no question. However, as you're reading this book all about the magnificence of the Inner Seasons and their potential to bring healing and balance to your life, I'm hoping that you're a tiny bit curious about exploring the Seasonal world more fully. Rest assured that while taking hormonal contraception, you can still access the Seasonal cycle by paying mindful attention to your moods and energy, as well as observing how you are affected by the lunar cycle. You'll find a link to download a moon chart in the Resources section.

Taking hormonal contraception can mask underlying hormonal imbalances, and not cure them. In their book *The Pill*, Jane Bennett and Alexandra Pope note:

We can see that through its profound hormonal impact the pill may also be interfering with the fundamental chemistry of who we are and what we can become.[5]

It's a common hope that taking the pill will 'fix' a period problem such as menstrual pain or premenstrual anxiety, for example. Sure, it can make it disappear, but it effectively masks the underlying physiological and psychological issues. For example, the pain might be caused by endometriosis, or by anxiety because of a trauma. As you've seen, the endocrine system is not a one-way street with oestrogen at one end and progesterone at the other. It's a complex junction of multi-levelled systems that affect *every* aspect of our mind, body, and being, so while we can be fairly certain we won't get pregnant while using contraception, we are also delaying our deeper healing.

As mentioned, the research into the side effects of hormonal contraception are mostly on younger women taking the pill. What does exist shows that the emotional side effects can be disturbing whatever our age, as suggested by these findings:

> *Hormonal contraceptive users, in contrast with non-users, were found to have higher rates of depression, anxiety, fatigue, 'neurotic' symptoms, sexual disturbances, compulsion, anger, and negative menstrual effects.*[6]

Does this list look at all familiar? It's *exactly* the same as the most common menopause symptoms. Another study showed that taking the pill had the effect of reducing libido altogether.[7] The studies into the emotional effects continued with one from the University of Copenhagen in 2017, which found a link between hormonal contraception and a higher risk of suicide.[8] Over a fifteen-year period they found that women taking hormonal contraceptives had up to triple the risk of suicide compared to women who had never taken hormonal contraception at all. In a previous study, the same group of researchers found that hormonal contraception was linked to depression, tracking one million Danish women aged between 15 and 34 over a period of thirteen years.[9] They discovered that women taking hormonal contraceptives were 70 per cent more likely to experience depression than those not taking hormonal contraceptives.

Taking the combined pill is not usually advised for the over-forties as there is an elevated risk of thrombosis and possible links with cardiovascular disease, breast and cervical cancer. [10]Your doctor is likely to advise you to change to the progesterone-only pill in this case. However, there are more subtle long-term physical effects, because hormonal contraception has been shown to deplete the body of key nutrients. Studies from the 1970s already showed a decline in glucose tolerance (which would account for weight gain while on the pill) and an apparent increase in the need for folate and vitamins C, B2 and B6 when using birth control.[11] More recently, it's been shown that levels of vitamin E, magnesium, selenium, and zinc are also depleted in women who are using birth control,[12, 13] and that some individuals also have associated issues with gut health.[14, 15] A younger body might not show the effect of this depletion for a while, but at perimenopause, when our system is highly sensitized anyway, we need all the nutrition we can possibly get.

Having read the chapters on food, gut health, and clearing out hormone disruptors, you are no doubt being super kind to yourself now, but if you are using hormonal birth control, you may be unwittingly *undoing* much of the love and care you have invested in. Is it worth it? Only you can decide. Life is complicated, and our situations and bodies infinitely varied, but being well informed about the bigger picture is vital. Knowledge is power.

Trying to find out what was going on with contraception in perimenopause, my colleague Andrea Clarke and I ran a small-scale survey. In our small sample of 40 respondents, 74 per cent of whom practised cycle awareness (as you might expect from our community), we saw an enormous range of experience. Most, at 67.5 per cent, used non-hormonal contraception such as condoms, withdrawal, copper coil or sterilization, and the remainder used the hormonal coil, and a small number were on the pill. Over all they rated their happiness with their contraception as a respectable 6.9 out of 10, which was a great surprise to me; I'd expected a catalogue of misery! What was even more fascinating was the huge variation in their experiences. The hormonal coil (which, anecdotally, can be savage) made bleeding much worse in one person, but reduced flow in another, thereby greatly improving her quality of life. Libido tanked because the coil became embedded in one person, yet libido went up after it was inserted in someone else; moods were worsened in some, improved in others, while some suffered more perimenopause symptoms in certain respects and barely noticed a thing in another, and others found no change in side effects during perimenopause at all. Repeat after me: there is no one-size fits all solution.

So how can we find the best solutions for ourselves? When researching contraception, we have to take a clear-eyed look at how we currently take care of ourselves, any possible health risks inherent with the various kinds of contraception, sensitivities to particular hormones, and how important it is for us to not get pregnant.

If you absolutely didn't want to risk any possibility of pregnancy, then hormonal contraception might be a good choice for you. But alongside finding the right method, it would be wise to have a look at your diet and stress levels, and to make sure that you are getting the maximum nutrients possible to support your body through the transition, and to see how you can build your emotional support systems to ensure good mental health. Above all, be prepared to be flexible and try different things until you find something that works for you in your situation.

If you were lucky enough to be practising menstrual cycle awareness during your menstruating years, you'll be winning. Having developed this sweet intimacy with yourself, you'll be in a good place to ride the changes of your menopause cycle and receive the gifts of the phases, and able to use methods such a natural family planning for contraception, where fertile windows are identified by temperature and cervical fluid.

PRACTICE
- Talk to your doctor or specialist about the benefits and risks of the different options of birth control.
- Talk to your partner/s about how they can be involved.
- Practise menstrual cycle awareness and listen to your body's needs.
- Journal into any emotional conflicts that might be playing out in your choices; for example, grief at the end of biological fertility, or what you think a family should look like, etc.

- Pay attention to your dreams: fertility is such a major issue and our dreams often speak to us loud and clear. Note them down in the mornings and return at a later time to catch the themes and messages.

Knowledge is power.

51 Lunar charting

If you don't have a regular period, you can chart your Inner Seasons by the moon instead of your menstrual cycle. Some people find that they are strongly influenced by the moon, noticing an intensity of feeling under the full moon and a more Wintery, inward sense in the days before the new moon. Australian fertility consultant Francesca Naish has gathered over forty years of clinical evidence on the lunar relationship with human fertility, which makes for fascinating reading.[1] Having had such a strong effect on a menstruating body, why would the moon's influence cease at menopause?

Personally, I feel only slightly affected by the full moon and am generally more aware of the influence of my 'birth moon'. The birth moon is the phase the moon was in on your date of your birth, which equates to the Inner Summer. You may find as I do, that the birth moon brings more expansiveness, and a more of a social focus. On the directly opposite side of the moon cycle, I am at my most low energy and inward, making it a time where I prioritize rest.

Check out Awen Clement's book *Moon Wise* for the low-down on natal moon phase cycles.[2] To find your own moon phase, just do an internet search for the moon phase on your date of birth; it couldn't be easier.

Even if you don't notice a regular pattern through the moon's phases, you can still use it to create rhythm and guidance in your life. Some like to treat the days before the new moon as their Inner Winter, taking a step back from the world to nourish themselves. To hold myself steady, I set intentions on the new moon, and then acknowledge and celebrate myself on the full moon, reflecting on how the intention has unfurled at the end of the cycle. This gives a lovely rhythm to my inner life, helping me to pace and care for myself in tune with the wider rhythms of the planet. There's more about intention setting in chapter 52. Just like menstrual charting to understand the Inner Seasons, charting with the moon is not about trying to conform to an expected pattern; it's an investigation into our own selves, to accept the subtlety of our own rhythms. We become an expert on ourselves.

PRACTICE

Charting your lunar month can be a chance to get super creative and use any medium you fancy. One friend paints a word each day on a stone, another doodles a little design alongside her words, a third makes a daily mandala. What would be pleasurable for you to do?

1. If you fancy, start charting your lunar cycle today, wherever you are, using a paper chart which can find in the Resources section.

2. If you prefer, design your own lunar chart on a computer and then print off two or more charts in one go, so you can continue smoothly into the next month.

3. Find out the moon phase for today, and put today's date in the appropriate space in the chart.

4. Just like charting with your cycle, note down things like:

- how you're feeling
- any pain
- sleep
- physical problems
- energy levels
- digestive problems
- dreams
- events like travel or other stressful situations
- what Inner Seasons are present for you
- dietary changes
- complementary therapy appointments
- supplements taken
- food cravings and appetite

Embrace the chaos: it's absolutely normal to not have a pattern.

I'm proud to be a lunatic.

MOON CHART

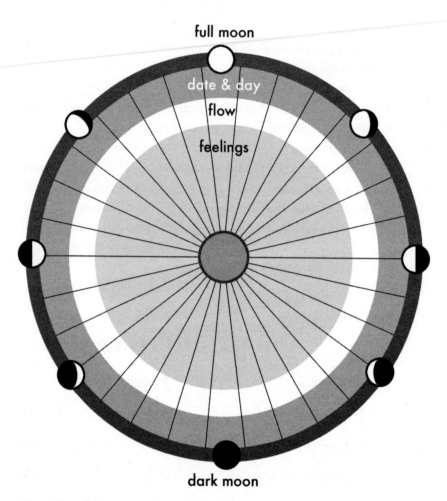

Created in collaboration with Leora Leboff

52 How to change

Everything starts with intention: making a cup of tea, going for a walk, finding a partner. First, we decide what we want, then we set about making it happen. Setting intentions from the heart can also be a gentle guide for qualitative shifts in your life, like feeling happier or more loving towards yourself. The process is no different from wanting a cup of tea: we just have to decide what we want and then refer our moment-to-moment decisions to this broader intention and let it guide our thoughts and actions. However, it is different from making a goal, which is based on wanting a specific outcome. An intention is about how you want to be in the present moment, which is particularly helpful while you're navigating the unpredictable menopause landscape and being assailed by challenging emotions, because it holds you steady. It is also a corrective – the call of the outer world is so loud, we need all the help we can get to stay close to our inner compass.

'I HAVE HAD AN INTENTION FOR A WHILE WHICH I KNOW HAS KICK-STARTED CHANGES IN MY LIFE. THAT IS THE INTENTION TO BE FREE AND ABLE TO FULFIL MY PURPOSE. I AM GETTING THERE AND FEEL THAT LOTS OF PROGRESS HAS BEEN MADE AND I AM CLOSE TO THAT GOAL.'

Sarah

The biggest game-changer for me in menopause was to hold an intention for more spaciousness in my life. It had been clear that I had to stop running around like a loony for some time – years in fact – but I just couldn't let go of trying to squeeze activity into every moment: kids, work, extra writing projects, training – there was no moment in the day that wasn't scheduled. A close friend was using intentions to create change in her life, so I thought I'd have a go.

It took a while to formulate the right words into something that I could commit to wholeheartedly. After trying a few intentions and tossing them out, 'spaciousness' felt good. I knew it was right, because I felt softer when I said it and my belly relaxed. It felt doable. Open enough to include all sorts of ways it might show up – from taking the time to cook really nice food, to allowing myself a day off once in a while. It was measurable because I could feel in my body the difference between the tightness of running around like a loony and the softness of having more space.

At first, I just wanted to create a little space between tasks – a simple thing you'd think, but my mind is always running on to the next thing and day after day I 'failed'. This is a very common event: by setting your intention, you somehow invite the universe to give you chapter and verse on how your patterns of behaviour are operating. You get to see where you're going wrong. I know – yay! But knowing that this was a thing allowed me to drop my judgement.

I knew that checking in with my intention morning and evening remained a healthy habit, and after a while I noticed that I wasn't failing so much as doing it differently; half-way through a task, I'd remember that I hadn't paused at the beginning, so I would take a breath. It became clear that I wasn't failing, but that the intention was working its way organically into my life without effort. I was slowing down. The changes seemed to happen magically of their own accord, without force, which had something to do with the way that the intention was held lovingly, softly even. But I also held on to it with a constancy that meant I continued to check in with it and to witness my changing behavioural patterns around filling up space. After a couple of years, I saw the quality of my life change from manic and ill to happy and well – with the added bonus of an enormous creative blossoming, excellent boundaries and the first sniff of Second Spring.

The beginning of any cycle is the natural time to set an intention, at the new moon, the start of your day, or period.

'THE INTENTION IS SET AT THE NEW MOON ANYWAY. IF YOU DON'T CHOOSE CONSCIOUSLY, THEN WHATEVER IS UNCONSCIOUS WILL BE SET AS YOUR INTENTION.'

Jane Hardwicke Collings, Women's Mysteries Teacher

In the Woman Kind community, we set our intentions at each new moon. Sometimes they're forgotten, sometimes they're brought to mind daily. Sometimes the very opposite happens and sometimes everything still turns out peachy. Regardless of the outcome, there is a power in letting our inner desires consciously direct the show.

We might as well choose, don't you think?

PRACTICE

- Journaling prompt: think of three people you admire and list the qualities you most value in them. See which quality resonates most strongly with you.
- To create your intention, take some quiet time out to reflect on the qualities you have listed in your journal, and on what gives you joy and where your values lie.

- Formulate an intention as a powerful statement in the positive, such as: 'I treat myself with respect' or 'I trust my body's wisdom'. You might want to drink less, for example, but setting the intention 'I treat myself kindly' will better help you to keep focused on your relationship with yourself, so you'll get so much more out of it.
- Once you've found something that feels good, bring it to mind before you get out of bed as you think of your day ahead. Before you go to sleep, review your day *with compassion*, noticing what tripped you up. Forgive yourself when things go pear-shaped, you are human after all. Shit happens.

Setting my intentions sets my reality.

53 You need your girlfriends

'WHEN I WAS RUNNING A CIRCLE
IN CORK, EACH WOMAN SAID,
"I THOUGHT I'D GONE MAD." IN
SEPARATING FROM EACH OTHER,
WE PLAY INTO THE IDEA THAT
IT'S MADNESS, BUT IN FACT,
IT'S A SUPERPOWER THAT IS ONLY
EVIDENT WHEN WE COME TOGETHER
AND SHARE OUR STORIES.'

*Uma Dinsmore-Tuli, activist and
author of* Yoni Shakti

Without good company, it's going to be a mighty bumpy ride. You are not going to be able to do this transition without your girlfriends. Friends are vital for our psychological wellbeing – they remind us of our goodness, give us courage and endless laughter – and at this point in our lives, we really start to see that good, trustworthy friends are rare jewels to be treasured. They last beyond marriages and illness, reminding us of who we are and why we are alive. There's even research that proves the blindingly obvious: friends will save your life. Having great friends reduces rates of heart disease, anxiety, and depression; they also improve your sense of purpose, happiness, self-worth, and confidence – and give you excellent gossip.[1,2]

'I'VE COMPLETELY CHANGED IN MY FORTIES. I FIND WOMEN RICH AND INTERESTING AND MEN'S BANTER VERY SHALLOW. I'VE REALLY CHANGED WHO I GRAVITATE TO AND ALSO FOUND JOINING A WOMEN'S CIRCLE INVALUABLE. I HAVE FOUR BROTHERS AND ALL FEMALE COMPANY WAS QUITE UNCOMFORTABLE FOR ME AT FIRST, BUT NOW I FIND IT NOURISHING. I WOULD CHARACTERIZE IT AS MEN HELP YOU TO RUN FAST WITH THEIR COMPETITIVE EDGE AND ENERGY, BUT WOMEN HELP YOU TO TAKE OFF AND FLY. THE SUPPORT I'VE HAD FROM WOMEN WHEN I'VE DONE COMEDY HAS BEEN PHENOMENAL.'

'Jodi'

Prioritize good relationships as part of your menopause medicine, starting close to home hang out with your mates or start a listening partnership (see chapter 24 for how to do this). There are an increasing number of menopause-friendly communities; for example, the Menopause Café, where you can eat cake and talk menopause in a confidential space. Other feminine-friendly, confidential spaces where you can really tell it how it is are Red Tents or the menopause-only equivalent, a Purple Tent.

If there's nothing around that really floats your boat, then start something yourself. I instigated a menopausal circle, the Fuck It Club, with a friend and have journeyed through menopause with six phenomenal women, squeezing hands all the way. We will be friends way beyond menopause and long into the future; the bond and trust we have developed is beautiful. Post-pandemic, we now have access to a range of flourishing online connections that we didn't have before; even if we feel isolated within our community, we can connect with like-minded people across continents and find our tribe that way.

'MOST OF MY CLOSE FRIENDS HAD GONE OR WERE GOING THROUGH PERI WITH ME. ONCE WE ALL REALIZED WHAT WAS GOING ON, WE DEEPLY UNDERSTOOD EACH OTHER'S FRUSTRATIONS, ANGER, THE LOSS OF CONTROL, THE ANXIETY. WE WERE ALL LEARNING AT THE SAME TIME, SO WE WERE ONLY ABLE TO SUPPORT EACH OTHER WITHIN THE LIMITS OF OUR OWN UNDERSTANDING.'

Sandra

Your superpower of discernment will help you view your friendships with renewed clarity. I often hear agonizing stories of conflicts where friends fall out, because the menopause is changing them in ways their friends can't handle. There's no getting away from seeing the truth of which friendships nourish you and where the vampires lurk in plain sight.

'I'VE DROPPED THE FRIENDS WHO HAVE BEEN A DRAIN ON MY ENERGY FOR YEARS AND FOCUSED ON MORE FUN FRIENDS WHO LIFT MY ENERGY AND WANT TO DANCE.'

Catherine

When energy is low and we're naturally feeling less social, it becomes obvious who we want to give our precious energy to and who we don't. If you're unsure about distancing yourself from a friend and need justification, check out the research on how toxic friendships shorten your life; it's about as bad for you as smoking.[3] It's not about quantity. Having a few wonderful friendships, rather than a lot of acquaintances, positively affects your bone health, as research organized by the Women's Health Initiative now shows:

> *'We found that bone loss is among the physiological stress responses more strongly related to the quality of social relationships than quantity.'*[4]

If you feel isolated and lonely within your community, don't despair: it's possible to find beautiful communities online where you can drop the exhausting mask of 'having to hold it all together' and just say it like it is, letting your inner experience speak. I recommend you use your excellent discernment to sniff out and avoid any fear-based, judgemental, advice-driven spaces. There are many safe communities for your experience to be honoured as you move from outrage at the disruption of Separation to the possibilities of new ways you could be. It's time to let go of the bullshit and find our own, better shit. That's the only conversation there is and, bloody hell, it's a good one.

PRACTICE

- Make a list of the people you consider your friends and reflect on how you feel when you see them. Are you full of life and good emotions, or left feeling depleted and exhausted?
- If you feel you don't have enough good interpersonal interactions, set an intention to reconnect with friends on a regular basis; don't let a day go by without telling someone you love them.
- You are fully entitled to disengage from outmoded, toxic friendships, no explanation required.

Find your tribe.

54 Love your bones

We think of our bones as static and dry: we take them for granted until we come to postmenopause, when the fears of osteoporosis arise, or, if you are unlucky, a small knock causes a big fracture.[1] In reality, our bones are a dynamic force. Research from Columbia University shows how bones play a part in turning on the fight-or-flight response in the body.[2] As soon as the brain recognizes danger, it tells the skeleton to fill the bloodstream with a hormone, osteocalcin, which turns on the response. The bones have a dynamic and complex relationship with the immune system, which is formed in the bone marrow where red blood cells are also created.[3] The bones are continuously growing too, so there's lots we can do to support good bone health now. It's worth knowing that bone density declines with lower oestrogen, but lower bone density *does not necessarily* lead to osteoporosis – just look at the lack of osteoporosis in Japan (see chapter 9).

In bodywork, the bones represent an aspect of our essential core self, our spirit, and using self-touch may help you to connect with the Second Spring you that would like to emerge. It's beautiful how the biological understanding of the bones leads naturally into our felt, energetic sense of being present on the earth.

Stress

Because the bones drive the fight-or-flight response by releasing the hormone osteocalcin, there is a strong link between osteoporosis and stress.[4,5] The easiest thing you can do to improve your bone health is find out how to relax and manage your stress better.

Food

Before you consider supplementation, have a look at what you're eating. Lani Simpson, whose bone-bible *The No-Nonsense Bone Health Guide* is stuffed with helpful information, advises that the quality of the food you take in is directly related to your bone density and overall bone quality.[6] She also recommends making good quality protein part of every meal and snack, alongside complex carbs such as oats, nuts, seeds, legumes, fruit, and veggies, especially dark green leafy ones, while also staying hydrated. The nice thing about hydration is that you can always fix it right now: go on, grab a glass of water – I am. Gut health plays a part too, and even the most immaculate diet won't be any use unless your digestion is on tip-top form to absorb all those lovely nutrients, so it's worth having a look back at chapter 29 on gut health if this is a concern. The other culprit in bone weakening is inflammation, so refer back to chapter 29 for more on inflammation if you're at risk.

Exercise

Doing weight-bearing exercise will help you build bone density.[7] High-impact exercise is most beneficial, meaning running, dancing, and jumping, etc. Yoga has shown good results too, with a daily 12-minute routine shown to reverse bone loss.[8] So far so practical, but what about tending to the spiritual life of our bones?

Body awareness

Have you chosen to be present in your bones? Can you really inhabit them? For such an essential aspect of our bodies, we give them precious little attention compared to our muscles or skin. Developing an awareness of your bones will help you to be grounded and present with yourself. The 'skin' of the bone, the periost, is also part of the fascia – the thin layer of connective tissue that surrounds and holds every organ, blood vessel, bone, nerve fibre, and muscle in place. You can feel the 'skin' of your bones, the periost, with your hands to start with, massaging the bones of the shin and ankle is a great place to start: then, when walking or moving, start to bring your attention to this deep part of your body and feel the difference it makes not only to your sense of presence and grounding, but to the whole body.

Soul

In *Women Who Run with the Wolves*, Clarissa Pinkola Estes tell the story of La Loba. It starts with an old woman who lives in a hidden place that everyone knows in their souls, but which no one has ever seen. The story goes on to describe how La Loba's task is to roam the country searching for wolf bones. She brings them back to her cave one by one and lays them out on the floor to make the wolf skeleton. Once all the bones are in place, she chooses the song to sing over the bones to give them flesh. The more she sings, the more the flesh fills and the creature breathes, until the floor of the desert shakes – and up jumps the wolf and runs away down the canyon, until it is transformed into a woman running free.

I love this story. It thrills me every time I read it because it narrates our soul's journey through menopause. Our task is to find the bones that inspire us and love them back into life, to sing them into being. The story tells us that we have the power to bring ourselves back to life, to make it through the dark of Winter.

PRACTICE
- Eat prunes: research has shown that eating five to six prunes a day reduces bone loss.[9,10]
- Get professional help: taking supplements is expensive and without careful research or guidance can result in expensive

wee or, at their worst, they may even contribute to your problems. It's worth investing in sessions with a qualified nutritionist to advise you, based on your individual needs. Or consult an experienced Functional Medicine practitioner, Functional Medicine being a biology-based approach that focuses on identifying and addressing the root cause of disease.

- Go to bed earlier, as short sleep is associated with bone loss.[11]
- A lovely practice to do by yourself, or even better, with a group of women, is to read the story of 'La Loba'. If you can't put your hands on a copy of *Woman Who Run with the Wolves*, search YouTube for footage of someone telling the story. Create an artwork in response – dance, paint, stitch, sing the story yourself.
- Put your hand on your shoulder and feel for your shoulder blade. Wiggle it around. Now find your shoulder joint, then imagining you could touch the bones of your arm, and massage down to your elbow, on through your forearm until you are touching the bones of your hand and fingers. When you've finished, compare one arm to the other and notice the difference between the two.

My bones are vitally alive and responsive to my attention.

55 The womb speaks

'THE WOMB IS CENTRAL TO ALL RITES OF PASSAGE IN A FEMALE BODY — MENARCHE, BIRTH AND MENOPAUSE. TO CONNECT WITH YOUR WOMB IS TO CONNECT WITH YOUR VERY ESSENCE. IF YOU WANT TO HAVE GOOD, INTIMATE SEX, CONNECT WITH YOUR WOMB.'

Jane Dancey, women's somatic health coach

If you fancy a short cut to the deep core of the menopause process, connect with your womb. If you don't have a womb, the energy is still there in the centre of the pelvic bowl. It is central to our physiological and psychological menopause process, because the womb holds the physicality of the Inner Seasons with its capacity to gather and release. Connecting with womb energy while you're menstruating, even if it is irregular, affirms your trust in the Seasons of life too. This capacity to gather and release also holds the key to our creative life, especially in Second Spring after our periods have stopped for good, when the energetic imprint of the Inner Seasons guides our creativity too. Connecting with our womb grounds us from the core of our being, into the earth so that we can better access our intuition and truth. Sceptical? Then have a look through some of the amazing physical and energetic qualities the womb possesses.

Sitting like a queen just above the pubic bone, behind the bladder, the womb is a truly awesome organ. Generally, we only think about her when she 'goes wrong' and gives us pain but, greatly underrated, she is the only organ to have the capacity to grow to twenty times her non-menstruating size and then shrink back down again. This is an astonishing kind of everyday magic. Did I mention that she can also grow a human? A human! I hope I never stop being astonished by this amazing ability. No wonder that the womb is ridiculed and shamed; this kind of power generates life of all kinds.

'IF YOU'VE GOT TO MENOPAUSE AND HAVEN'T TAKEN THE TIME TO LISTEN IN BEFORE, YOUR WOMB IS LIKELY TO BE SCREAMING AT YOU FOR ATTENTION. TRUST ME, WHAT YOU'LL FIND OUT ABOUT YOURSELF AND IT WILL BE WELL WORTH THE TIME AND EFFORT.'

Andrea Clarke, Holistic Pelvic Care® therapist

More or less every month over a woman's menstruating years, the womb ripens and fills, and if there's no pregnancy, releases her lining sweetly. An ace magic trick! Or more commonly known as a curse. Our bleeds have been loaded with more shame than any other bodily function. Patriarchy has properly shafted her capacity to renew herself and give us access to all the Seasons' gifts.

In an average woman, the womb will double in weight from 2oz in a young woman mid-cycle to 8oz menstrual weight, which is carried by the ligaments. The ligaments, also made of connective tissue, are sometimes held tightly or unevenly so that the womb leans backwards or forwards, or to one side or the other, making it trickier to release fully when the period comes. Once again, our modern, sedentary life serves us badly in this, with prolonged stretches of sitting restricting blood flow and creating more stagnation in the pelvic bowl.

With the process of menopause, the womb will shrink down to an almost pre-pubescent size, mirroring the many ways in which we return to our teen-self in Second Spring. Without the regular release of periods, we may need to find other ways to consciously let go in menopause.

'INTENSE HEAT AND PRESSURE, THE COMPRESSION OF OUR UTERUS, THE OPPORTUNITY FOR CHANGE, GIVES US A DIAMOND OF OUR OWN. A BRIGHT, SHINING LIGHT RIGHT IN OUR CENTRE WHICH CAN BE A LIGHT TO SHINE FOR THOSE WHO CAN RECOGNIZE IT AND A BRILLIANCE TO ILLUMINATE OUR OWN LIVES EACH AND EVERY DAY.'

Hilary Lewin, women's health therapist[1]

Energetic womb space

'THE WOMB IS TRANSMITTER OF
VITAL INFORMATION REGARD-
ING PHYSICAL AND EMOTIONAL
STATUS. A CREATIVE ORGAN, NOT
JUST FOR MAKING BABIES BUT TO
MANIFEST THE LIFE YOU LONG FOR.'

Hilary Lewin, women's health therapist

When talking about the energetic presence of the womb, I'm referring to the energy that fills the pelvic bowl, which exists whether we have a womb or not. This is the energy of grounding and our connection to the earth, and of creativity and sexuality. It's the energy of the Feminine principle (big F) and this is where we can get into a tangle because the way you and I understand 'Feminine' is going to be vastly different, depending on the messages you were given about being a woman. If you have a problem with using the term Feminine, try changing the language to 'earth', 'energy', 'flow' or something else that reduces the charge enough to enable you to explore this quality more easily.

Feminine principle is something other than how we experience being a woman. It's the cyclical flow of the Inner Seasons, the capacity to receive, to connect with the earth, and contain and then to nourish and release. It means having the capacity to access knowing about what will nourish and what will not, in the biggest sense imaginable: relationships, food, creative projects, everything. Connecting with the Feminine principle will give you a big chunk of self-knowledge, whatever gender orientation you feel closest to. But these are all just empty words on a page; to find out what your version of the Feminine is *really* like you have to dive into connection with your womb-space to experience it.

I can illustrate this with a bit of my story. I was a total airhead. I loved to dream, fly, float, and drift and get carried away with ideas to the extent that my overexcitement used to scare people. And as for grounding? That was *sooo* boring! Who the hell wanted to do that? Except, of course, getting carried away meant I couldn't really be present, stay in relationship, or follow projects all the way through.

This imbalance continued until I got into abdominal massage and started to connect with my pelvis. I have to say, that if you'd have told me to connect with the Feminine at that point in my life, I would have shot off like a rocket, I held it in such negative regard. By using the Self-care Abdominal Massage that focused on my pelvis and building awareness there, without even trying, I started to ground and truly connect with the earth in a way that just wasn't available to me before.

By engaging with the Inner Seasons, even while my fertile years were waving goodbye, I started to get comfortable with the Feminine *on my own terms*, without the toxic messages I continue to receive from my culture about what that means. For example, I finally began to let go of dressing to try to demonstrate a culturally approved 'nice', 'female' silhouette and began wearing what made me happy instead. Also I started dropping being 'capable' and 'supportive' in favour of following the flow of my Inner Seasons.

Another example is of a client who came to see me because she had fibroids. She had followed a lifelong career in healthcare, lovingly tending the vulnerable, but by connecting with her womb realized that this work had left no room for her own creative passions, which she had longed to engage with. What is required is to be present to the quality of the energy of the pelvic bowl and the Inner Seasons as they present to you. The Feminine is there at your door, giving you the answers.

Holistic Pelvic Care® visionary Tami Lynn Kent speaks eloquently about the value of the pelvic bowl. In her book *Wild Feminine*, Tami frames this around 'women', but these processes are available to all of us, regardless of gender:

> *'Encircled by pelvic bones, round and smooth, the root of the female body is like a bowl. Here in the womb, a woman will find the energy she holds for herself and for mothering her creations. For centuries, women have been the bowl. They have been the basket makers, weaving containers that held food and water just as their bodies held the energy of the children and home. In modern settings, a woman's body still holds or releases energy from the root.'[2]*

Interviewee Samantha's menopause experience brought them dramatically back into contact with their womb, which healed a life-long issue. They shared with me how not feeling connected with their womb had made them feel that 'they didn't belong here'. The issues with food and alcohol had been an attempt to fill the void that they'd felt from the ribs downwards. Menopause brought awareness dramatically into the belly and womb through a shamanic experience, bringing the gift that they could now reconnect with their own, birth-given wisdom. They explained:

> *'The void is still there but it is now my connection to the universe: if I want to get to the truth of something or connect with a person, I do it from my lower gut and womb.'*

PRACTICE

- Use the Womb Journey Meditation (see pages 147–148) or the Self-Care Abdominal Massage (see pages 74–76) to explore your womb and your relationship to the Feminine, whatever this means to you.

Define your own Feminine.

56 Your 'downstairs' department speaks

Listen to your body. Sounds like an easy thing to do, doesn't it? Tiredness requires rest. Twitchiness requires movement. The body speaks all right, especially in menopause, loud and clear in the language of pain, of crappy posture and cramped movement; but bridging the gap from there to a conscious understanding can be challenging.

Carl Jung reminds us:

'Bodily illness can affect the psyche; for psyche and body are not separate entities, but one and the same life.'[1]

Having spent upwards of twenty-five years of my life trying to listen to my body and helping others to listen to theirs, I know it's not always simple to access body wisdom, but I am *always* knocked out by the information that shows up. When we can truly listen and hear what our body asks of us and follow through with our actions, healing happens on so many levels. Resting when we are tired, for example, not only restores our own energy, but helps us to soften and connect with those around us, have enough energy to set firm boundaries, plan treats, and stay on track with our intentions. It seems that our bodies know already what is required and the biggest part of the piece might be learning to trust that. There's no need to look elsewhere for answers.

'THERE'S A SENSE OF BEING MORE
WILLING TO LISTEN TO WHAT I NEED
TO DO IN THE MOMENT. I WAS
GOING TO CREATE SOMETHING ON
MONDAY BUT MY BRAIN STUCK TWO
FINGERS UP AT THAT, THERE WAS
NO WAY I COULD DO IT, SO I TOOK
THE DAY OFF. I'D NEVER HAVE DONE
THAT BEFORE.'

Annya, acupuncturist and mindfulness teacher

I had been practising bodywork for more than twenty-five years and a big part of my identity was bound up in being a therapist, when my hands started to speak to me. They swelled and stiffened to the point that I was losing my ability to hold saucepans and open jars. I had been aware of the pain for some time but the metaphor of 'losing my grip' came almost instantly to mind when I found I couldn't open a jar of pickles one day. And I love pickles! I realized I had literally 'lost my grip' on who I was. If I wasn't this helpful therapist person, then who was I? I had to absolutely let go of that role before I could move on.

To 'mind the gap' and surrender into the possibility that I did not know who I was, while terrifying, opened the door to a wider range of possible futures and ways of being. I still wasn't properly listening until I decided to devote twenty minutes to actually having a conversation with my hands. Like having any kind of mindful listening, it required particular conditions. Quiet, curiosity, open awareness, and parking the judgements outside the door. Only then could the question be asked: 'What is it that I need to know?'

My hands began to move softly as I watched them, and with my attention staying with the sensation as best I could, I mindfully observed what was happening and my thoughts as they arose. I explored trying to grip tightly, being still, and soft movement – all the while holding on to the question: 'What is it I need to know?' What I noticed was how exhausting the tightness was and how that wore me out; and that it was the rigidity with which I was holding on to my role as a therapist that was the problem, rather than just the physical movement involved in the work. There was a noticeable easing in my symptoms that day, as though having felt heard, my hands could let go a little, maybe even trust me more. Over the following days, the more I thought about it, and the kinder I was to my hands, the clearer it became. I had to stop.

Our bodies communicate to us in their own unique ways. You might receive the information in a dream, by movement, or being still, by journaling, drawing or creating, alone or with a therapist, or through visualization. You might connect better with a gentle touch. It might come super fast and clear, or the understanding might grow over a longer time period. Sometimes you must hold your attention on the body part; sometimes you have to go and do something completely unrelated before the information arrives. The next time you have pain or a symptom that is bothering you, commit to having a mindful moment and ask, 'What is it I need to know here?' and you will be surprised at what your body has to say. Poet Kai Seidenberg describes this process beautifully in her poem 'Ask Your Body':

Ask your body
how it wants
to move,
and allow it
to answer
in its own way
and time.

Look past
the mind,
that quick and
clever pupil
in the front row
who invariably
jumps up
and yells out
an answer. [2]

PRACTICE

You might like to use a Circle process (see chapter 16) to understand what your body is saying.

The Self-Care Abdominal Massage (see pages 74–76) is also an excellent way to get in touch with your body's wisdom.

Take some time to reflect on what you need to feel connected with yourself: is it better alone or held by a therapist, silence or music, movement or stillness. Perhaps you like to journal, draw or sing?

Listening to your body requires some structure to hold you, as well as the flexibility and openness to receive the information. Take a look at this checklist to create a nourishing environment for yourself:

- commit a specific amount of time
- ensure a peaceful environment
- get comfy and relax
- make it safe
- let go of expectations and judgements
- be still
- ask: 'What is it I need to know here?'
- stay as present in your body as you can

Be your own guru.

57 We need a gap year

The natural withdrawal from everyday duties sometimes pulls us away entirely, either by accident or design. Clients report how being made redundant or furloughed during the pandemic can evoke a secret sigh of relief that we no longer have to pretend we care about 'that stuff', once the initial shock passes. As in all menopause health issues, the racial and economic inequality in our society widens the divide between the privileged and the marginalized. It's apparent in the different symptoms we experience and the take-up of HRT, but even more so in the possibility of dropping work or family commitments. Menopause is often described as a 'women's issue', but it's more accurate to say that it's a social justice issue.

In an ideal world, every menopauser would have the right to on-demand, state-sponsored time out. In one Australian study, a quarter of menopausal women wanted to take at least some time off.[1] Some degree of retreat from the world is an essential part of the Surrender phase and allows us to rest and heal. The yearning is strong for activities with no purpose and no goal, unburdened with anyone else's needs but your own; drifting, dreaming, gazing, pottering, and, of course, sleeping. There is such a ravenous hunger for space in Surrender, that sometimes it feels that no mountain range, no beach, could ever be big enough.

'I DIDN'T HAVE A BUSY LIFE OR WORK TWELVE-HOUR SHIFTS, BUT WHAT I REALLY WANTED WAS SIX MONTHS OFF.'

'Suze'

Artist and yoga teacher Frances Lewis coined the term 'menopause gap' when she left her regular life:

'Friends offered me space to live in ... I decided not to get out of bed in the morning until I felt a sense of self-love ... I learned to rest and allow support and let my action come out of rest that is naturally arising rather than pushing or grasping ... Not follow a rigid pattern but to rest when I'm tired, to do things when I felt enthusiasm.'[2]

The uprising of creative energy this brought resulted in a beautiful book, *The Divine Dance in the Sacred Landscape of Britain*.[3]

When you can't take time out

Unfortunately, in the real world, gap years are hard to come by. So what can we do when we can't get away?

- Consciously claim time out for yourself − even five minutes will help. A cup of tea, a walk, sinking your toes into grass, or just taking a conscious step away from your life is wonderful medicine.
- Some chuck their 'big' jobs in and exchange these for something that will let them coast for a while.

- Holding the tension between your inner and outer life is a prime menopausal skill. It takes dedication to hold the importance of your inner life, especially where you have to work in the real world. One way is to look busy but do less, acting as if you are in the 'ordinary' world – where in fact your inner needs to do less are primary.
- Is it possible to live more simply, reduce out-goings and do less? What could you let go of doing? Perhaps your house need not be so tidy or so clean? Maybe the kids could make their own way to their activities? Maybe you don't have to cook quite so often? What tasks can you delegate? They may not be done as well or as efficiently as you do them but reducing your expectations of yourself can be enormously liberating.
- Perhaps you could commit to a period of time where you just do less, telling your friends and family that you're on a semi-gap year and normal service will be resumed soon?
- Dreaming of a tropical retreat? Why not recreate it at home by designating a special space as your menopause nest? It could be a corner of your bedroom or living room, a place in your garden or in nature, somewhere you can go to let your mind drift and hang up your 'do not disturb' sign.
- Pottering is also an excellent at-home menopause gap.
- Slow your pace.

Midway through my menopause, after tying myself in knots trying to resolve the conflict between earning a living and my physical and mental health, I began to see that I would have to let go. Stop work completely to be able to see what needed to happen next. I acknowledge my privilege in that I found that once I had fully committed to letting it all go, the finances fell into place to make sure that the bills were paid, and all would be well. This was my Surrender.

Do you have to take time off from work and/or family to Surrender in menopause? No. In a perfect world, should every woman have the opportunity to do so if she wants to? Hell, yes!

Embarking on this six-month sabbatical was exquisitely sweet for me.

Every task – from washing up to cleaning the loo – filled me with a radiant joy because I was *choosing* to do it. I had a few rules:

- only do stuff that was pleasurable, or reframe, or press delete if not
- all thoughts of work/identity were forbidden until a month before the end
- to arrest my inner critic and hold her hostage for the duration
- reject anything goal-orientated

Letting go is hard to do, it's where the unknown lurks, like the troll under the Billy Goats Gruffs' bridge. Here's another menopause gap experience, this time from Andrea Clarke:

> *Letting go of the 'doing' was profoundly difficult. What I love though, is that my menopause gap gave others permission to do the same and it started to become a 'thing'. One day it will just be another recognized part of this transitional journey – how exciting is that?*

This period was a time of deep creativity for me. From a place of having no goals and just enjoying the process, I explored new avenues and mediums – and came up with a whole new healing/art form/activism in The Pants of Empowerment. This project allows people to access the creative crucible of their pelvic bowl, and based on this experience, I made them bespoke pants: wearable art. Their beautiful stories of real-life compromise, riches, and sexuality are published to inspire others. I drew, painted, and re-engaged with textiles and made clothes again, just as I had when I was a teenager.

'I TOOK THREE MONTHS LEAVE
FROM WORK AND PUT MYSELF BACK
TOGETHER. THAT REALLY HELPED.'

'Marie'

PRACTICE

- Practise saying *no* to things; try small ones at first. If you need help, see chapter 59.
- Make yourself a 'do not disturb' sign to put on your door.
- Delegate tasks.
- Journaling prompt: if you had a day where your fairy godmother gifted you a menopause gap, what would you do with it? What would 1 per cent of this look like?
- Take 30 minutes of time from your day and only do what is pleasurable for you; give yourself permission to let go of any other goals or outcomes.

Only do things that are pleasurable; otherwise reframe or delete them.

58 Menopause at work

Though women are still paid less on the whole than men, we're better educated than ever before and more of us are working for longer than at any other time. The fastest growing demographic, 75 per cent to 80 per cent of perimenopausal and menopausal woman are in work, and there will be many more postmenopausal women in work in the years to come.[1] A decade ago, women in the UK could claim their state pension at the age of 60, but by the time you are reading this, it is predicted to be 66 and rising to 67. Change is happening, evidenced by the rash of menopause policies being celebrated in major companies across all sectors, but the awareness is slow to percolate through to the actual shop floors and desks of the people who need it.

Time taken off work because of menopausal symptoms still causes a loss of 14 million working days annually. This lack of support costs businesses dearly. One in three menopausal women consider leaving their jobs or don't take senior roles, and that is an expensive mistake for businesses. The true cost of recruitment is estimated to be equal to or more than the annual salary of a post, once the expenses have been factored in relating to advertising, agency fees, lost productivity, and catching-up time etc. And it's not just a financial loss: remember how older brains see the bigger picture and can spot failures in the system? Add to this the menopausal gift of discernment, and companies risk losing some of their greatest assets when they do not support people through this transition.

Even in the health sector, where you'd think they were better informed, it was found that:

A lack of support during the menopause has led some female doctors to consider reducing their hours, stepping back from senior roles, including doctor partnerships, or quitting the profession altogether.[2]

Half of those surveyed were afraid to talk to their line manager about their menopause. This in an industry that *surely* should be well informed about gynaecological health.

The UK Equality Act 2010 protects people from discrimination for their gender, age, and disability at work, so that everyone is meant to be treated equally in terms of opportunities and pay. This means you should not lose out on training, promotion or pay because your employer has not supported you through menopause. There have been cases where people have successfully claimed discrimination because they were sacked due to menopause issues. For example, a 2012 tribunal held that direct sex discrimination had occurred when British Telecommunications failed to treat an employee's menopause in the same way as other medical conditions when applying its performance management policy. Another case in 2018 was successfully prosecuted under the disability act. Supporting menopause makes good business sense[3].

Amongst the army of menopausal people running the country, brain fog is the most commonly reported issue, affecting performance and deadlines and undermining confidence. This is not helped by a lack of sleep, making an 8.30am breakfast meeting a terrifying prospect, especially when you're worrying about it at 4am. Hot flushes cause fluster and embarrassment:

> *'I used to sit in meetings with a bank of fans ranked in front of me; I went and told my boss that I wasn't sleeping and that the health issues would pass. That job ended in a redundancy but I have never been sure how much of that was to do with menopause.'*
>
> *'Supriya'*

> *'I found myself in floods of tears because of a small mistake that shouldn't have bothered me, I felt like I'd be taken over, possessed even!'*
>
> *'Mell'*

The public service union Unison adds:

> *Many women are being driven from the workplace because they find that adapting problematic symptoms around inflexible work expectations is just too difficult. Others may find that managing symptoms mean they miss out on promotions and training, reduce their hours, lose confidence in the workplace and see their pay levels drop, all contributing to a widening gender pay gap.[4]*

Not to mention that half of us are paddling our duck feet frantically under the water, working in our own time to catch up with things. The most pressing problem for both individuals and for companies is the crisis in confidence resulting from menopause being regarded as an embarrassment that is best ignored.

The way menopause is handled almost entirely depends on how approachable your line manager is and this is why company-provided training and awareness is essential to create an open and accommodating environment for conversations about menopause, in the same way as any other health condition, so that everyone understands that menopause is normal for woman as well as others who identify as trans and non-binary.

Marks & Spencer led the way in 2003 by introducing the right to request flexible working and dedicated menopause advice on their staff website[5]. Nottinghamshire Police introduced their menopause policy by issuing guidance to managers saying they could consider requests from women who needed to adjust their uniform or their working hours. Among the practical support, it recommended access to private areas where people could: 'rest temporarily, cry or talk with a colleague before they can return to their workspace' according to the *Guardian* newspaper, evoking visions of comfy sofas, chocolate and abandoned truncheons rolling across the floor.[6] These are provisions that will benefit 'civilians' as well as those who are menopausal.

Menopause awareness goes beyond the people suffering symptoms; after all, non-menopausers will have colleagues, partners, mothers, friends, and sisters who experience it, and who also need support. My interviewee Helen created a menopause policy in her electrical contracting business, JHP Electrical Services:

Running a firm with family values, I wanted menopause to be on a par with anyone experiencing IVF, a bereavement or any health issue, so that it was dealt with sensitively and compassionately.

Bringing a degree of cyclical awareness to the workplace will not only benefit the menstruators and menopausers, but everyone. Understanding that we *all* need to take our foot off the gas in our Autumns and Winters makes for a healthier team, with fewer absences and burnouts. If the gifts of the Seasons can also be utilized intelligently by managers, imagine harnessing all that discernment – it would save a fortune in business consultants!

Training should ensure that everyone at all levels of the company gets clear information about what menopause is, so staff can confidently have conversations about how they can get support for their symptoms.[7] Where it's not possible to confidently approach a line manager, the next point of contact within HR or occupational health should be clearly defined. Training should also include awareness that menopause can affect the trans and non-binary folk too and that race and disability also come into play in accessing appropriate services. The unions all have great guides to setting up policy but the best way is not to make assumptions; instead, ask the people you're trying to engage what they might need. Beyond the training and an open, compassionate culture, it can be an idea to:

- Allow time and provide space for peer networks.
- Record absences as an ongoing health issue, rather than a short-term absence.
- Offer counselling for the effects on mental health.
- Make flexible and home working available on request.
- Be able to change workspace location within the workplace.
- Provide private 'break-out' spaces available for a breather.
- Allow for privacy in accessing toilets.
- Make ventilation available in the workspace.

If you would like training or ideas for creating an open, menopause-friendly workplace there are recommendations in the Resources section at the end of the book.

Above all, research and insight director Rebekah Boston recommends being honest and upfront about your symptoms: after all, saying you're fine when you're not looks super suspicious and will cause more tension for you and your team.

PRACTICE

Beyond instigating training and starting conversations, how can you bring a dose of Autumn and Winter sensibility to the endless Summer of the workplace? Here are some suggestions.

- Employ your menopausal gifts of discernment and not-give-a-fuckery to rigorously prioritize what is important for you to do, and forget or delegate the other tasks.
- Take regular breaks. Walk round the office, spend time alone in the loo, enjoy a complete cycle of breathing, a short meditation or breath app – anything that brings you back to yourself.
- Combat brain fog by being a list maniac and preparing thoroughly for important presentations.
- Ask for help from people you trust: engage colleagues, mentors, peer groups, managers or HR in the discussion about menopause and tell them what you need.
- Consider instigating a peer-lead network for menopause; anecdotally, I hear that it dramatically reduces the number of warnings for underperformance and sick leave.

You and your symptoms are worthy of care and kindness.

59 The power of NO to say YES to yourself

'YOU SEE THAT THE EMPERORS'
ARSE IS OUT AND NAKED. WE
HAVE A POWERFUL CAPACITY TO
SEE WHAT IS ABSURD ABOUT THE
FORMER WAYS OF DOING THINGS.'

Uma Dinsmore-Tuli, activist and author of Yoni Shakti

Have you ever met someone for coffee because you didn't want to upset them? Gone to a party because your friend needed support, though you were already knackered? Let someone 'pick your brains' when you were super busy? There's not a person alive who hasn't. We've been encouraged since we were girls to keep other people happy as a way of being valued, and to look after other peoples' needs before our own. When we have abundant energy, the slight imbalance in the exchange is negligible. But the great wake-up call of menopause brings an end to 'seconding' ourselves, assisted by Autumn and Winter's gifts of truth-telling and knowing.

'THE "TAKING NO SHIT" OF AUTUMN
IS SPREADING SLOWLY INTO THE
OTHER SEASONS.'

Julia

Maybe it's the lowered oestrogen levels that make us less accommodating or maybe it's just because we're knackered. Either way, the result is remarkable clarity about what you are willing to put up with. Where once you smiled and nodded in the face of nonsense, now you call it out. Bullshit detectors are set to high.

'DID I TELL YOU ABOUT THE MOMENT WHEN
MY HUSBAND WAS PLANTING A GOOSE-
BERRY BUSH AND I QUITE CLEARLY REAL-
IZED I DIDN'T WANT TO GROW ANYTHING
MORE WITH THIS MAN? WHEN HE FINALLY
LEFT, ONE OF THE FIRST THINGS I DID WAS
PULL UP THE PLANT. IT WAS A MOMENT
OF CLARITY HIGHLIGHTING MY OWN
BULLSHIT RE THE RELATIONSHIP AND MY
PLACE IN THE WORLD.'

Cryn

Low energy brings infinite clarity about what is worth doing and what is not. Surrender brings us to a place where we have learned to put our self first. Even those of us who, like my pre-menopausal self, are addicted to dithering now find ourselves settling on a single binary question: will this nourish or deplete me? In the choppy seas of menopause, even joyful things can be depleting – the interesting job that requires a long journey, or a project that's just too big altogether. Fun stuff can be too much because we're more sensitive to stress. Things that used to be a doddle might not be within your capability now. This is not a failure but about right timing – it is the yin Season and to emerge fully in Second Spring we must prioritize rest. Sharon explained:

> *Strong boundaries have now become essential, as opposed to before, when they were "nice to have". Almost a matter of life and death. The distinction between "have to" and "want to" and "need to" and "don't" is crystal clear.*

In the Winter of our menopause, our intuition is much more accessible to us than at other times. We 'know it in our waters', as a 'gut reaction'. We tend to think that our brains are the rulers of the body. But while they're busy worrying about global warming and the creep of right-wing extremism across the world, the gut is quietly in charge. It possesses an area of specialized nerves as large and complex as the brain, and activity in the solar plexus is, in fact, sending signals to the brain and not the other way around; in other words, *the belly is telling the brain what to think*. Your gut reactions are literally running the show and are a brilliant resource to tap into. Learning to trust our guts and to feel into our responses when we're invited to do something is an open doorway to our discernment.

Just say no

'I HAVE ALWAYS FOUND SAYING NO
VERY DIFFICULT. BUT NOW I FIND
IT FALLS OUT OF MY MOUTH BEFORE
I'VE HAD CHANCE TO CONSIDER
HOW THEY WILL RECEIVE THE
NEGATIVE ANSWER.'

Caroline

It's one thing feeling it in your guts, but taking action is quite another. One of the most awesome of menopausal superpowers is the power of NO. It will set you free to dabble in all sorts of more pleasurable things like resting, pottering, and dreaming. This superpower is birthed from a marriage of Autumnal truth-telling and fatigue. If you've ever taken on more than you should and wished you hadn't, this is your classroom for learning to say no. Here are some wonderful ways of saying no I have learned from my clever friends:

- *'On this occasion, I have to say no'*: suggests regret and the possibility of future kindness, while avoiding having to make excuses as to why you can't.
- *'I'd rather not'*: brilliant combination of politeness and finality.
- *'Thanks for thinking of me, but I have enough on right now'*: gratitude plus vague excuse.
- *'Not this time, thank you'*: softening the no by holding the door open.

Top tips for saying no

- Start with a compliment.
- If you're struggling, buy yourself time – say you'll have a think and get back with an answer later.
- Smile when you say it.
- You don't need to explain why.
- Trust your guts: if your stomach gets tight at the thought of the task, say no.
- You can say no more than once.
- Check the task against your intention to be kind to yourself.
- Change the subject or excuse yourself afterwards.
- It gets easier the more you practise.

This doesn't just concern menopause either. For any project to come to its full potential, we have to say no to other things.

PRACTICE
- Say no to something or someone today.

No is a complete sentence.

60 You will be asked to let go some more

How long does this take? When is Second Spring coming, please? Can this finally be over now?

I'm just dropping in here to remind you that you're doing just fine, you're not getting this wrong, not at all. Even if we go into menopause more or less consciously, we know that we have to let go. We can do this, right? In every conversation I've ever had about menopause, I hear that we are asked to let go again and again and again. No matter how much we know, how much awareness, and how we think we've got it nailed, menopause is *meant to be an undoing*. It is messy and requires us to be undone. Menopause is *fierce!*

> 'I'M UNRAVELLING, I CAN'T FINISH
> ANYTHING AT ALL!'
>
> '*Jo*'

We take a step back from work, but then injure ourselves so we can't do anything. We let go of our tendency towards perfection, but are challenged by a family member in crisis, and so on. There's always another level to let go of. It is terrifying. We've learned the tough lesson that we have to be in control, to push and 'make shit happen' all our lives. We have learned *not* to trust in the cyclical swing of our inner and outer worlds, but now we are forced to listen, and we are humbled.

Our coping mechanisms are unravelling like a hand-knitted sweater: the more we pull at it, the more it comes undone. The armour of coping mechanisms that have kept us from feeling lost, unlovable, unworthy have passed their sell-by date. Life is short. It is time to reclaim the love and belonging that you came into the world with, and to allow new things to *come through you*. In her essay 'Midlife Unraveling', Brené Brown has this down and perfectly describes the fierce urgency of menopause as it nips at our heels[1]. Like the sheep in the movie *Babe*, we try to run away shouting, 'Wolf! Wolf!' – but unlike the sheep, we can't outrun menopause. She is too fierce in her pursuit.

'IT IS EXTRAORDINARILY LIBERATING, AND IN THE PROCESS OF BEING HUMBLED, FREEDOM EMERGES.'

Alexandra Pope, co-founder of Red School

This is freedom from pushing, so things can start to emerge *through* us. Perhaps this is the major difference between before and after transition: a pre-menopausal woman believes she can make shit happen, a post-menopausal woman allows the shit to come through.

PRACTICE
- Do nothing
- Or if you want to do something, lie down and practise one of the yoga nidras.

It is enough for me to be
here, in this moment.

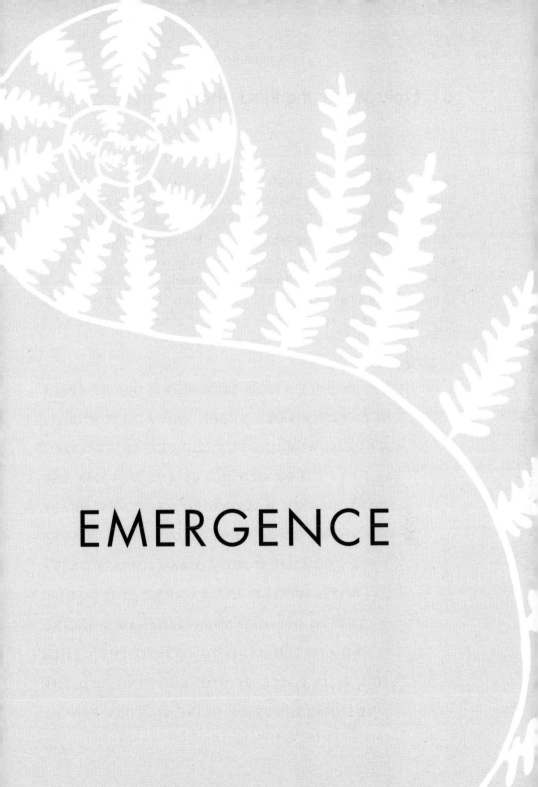

EMERGENCE

61 Emergence: the third phase of menopause

During Surrender, the new shoots of possibilities, energy, and ideas emerge imperceptibly, announcing the next phase: Emergence. It's such a relief to experience new life after the long Wintery retreat, that your impulse will be to rush out and make stuff happen. It was certainly true for me. But the days of Emergence are extraordinarily tender times; think of little lettuce seedlings tricked into growth by early spring sunshine, only to be frozen by a late frost: we still need protection. It is too early to go out there. The core around which everything rotates in Emergence is: 'What the hell do I do with the rest of my life?'

'EMERGENCE FEELS LIKE BEING IN THE SPACE BETWEEN AN OLD SHAPE AND A NEW ONE. IT CAN FEEL WOBBLY, VULNERABLE AND PAINFUL AS I LET GO OF OLD HOPES AND DREAMS AND STAND NAKED, WAITING FOR THE NEW SHAPE AND VISION TO BE REVEALED. IT IS A TENDER TIME AND IT IS GOOD TO BE COMPASSIONATE WITH MYSELF AND PATIENT AND NOT TO TRY TO USE OLD STRATEGIES OF FORCING AND CONTROLLING TO GET TO THE OTHER SIDE. IT IS PLACE OF NOT-KNOWING AND THE VULNERABILITY OF BEING IN THAT PLACE.'

'Mel'

We have let go of what wasn't working, the bits and bobs that kept us small. We've been humbled to the vulnerability of not knowing. What's next? Who do I want to be when I grow up? And how the hell do I do that? This phase enables us to try out scenarios, to dream, fantasize, to long for things. Perhaps to live next to the sea, write those poems, or train to be a teacher. This dreaming can allow all the lovely oxytocin to wash through you and soothe your system, reducing stress and balancing your hormones. Daydreaming is an actual medicine for menopause! In real life there will be compromises and challenges and conflict, so why not enjoy the fantasy while you can? All top-performing athletes use visualization as part of their tools for achievement because it talks directly to our subconscious.

Paradoxically, alongside this sometimes angsty quest for the next step, is also resistance to emerging. Now that we're finally tucked up in our Winter Surrender-mode, we find it so cosy that thought of returning to the 'out there' world is scary. Quite often we feel the pull of opposing forces between the soul-quest to express our being in the world and a sense of delicious laziness once we have relaxed into our Winter.

The end of your period is the Seasonal equivalent of Emergence in menopause. It's a time that is often skipped over as we rush back out to get on with our to-do list, but it is extraordinarily tender. Being gentle with ourselves at this time by easing ourselves back into the world is an act of deep self-kindness that can affect the whole of the next menstrual cycle, and so it is in menopause.

In Emergence we are required to trust the process, hold the charge between inner and outer, and receive inspiration and energy. This phase is often skipped over because it's such a relief to have a little more energy again, and finally feel better. The temptation is to rush out of the menopause cave and *do loads of stuff.* Coming back to our butterfly analogy, it has to emerge slowly from the chrysalis and dry its wings in the sun before it can fly away.

PRACTICE

- Enjoy the Yoga Nidra for Emergence on pages 317–320.
- Give yourself time to dream into the possibilities your life might hold; and let yourself indulge and enjoy the warmth of your fantasies without judgement.
- Ponder on what you're afraid of losing if you really got what you long for: this fear might be holding you back.

What do I want to be when I grow up?

Yoga Nidra for Emergence

This nidra will give you about 15 minutes of deep rest. Find a cosy space where you can recline undisturbed, with all the cushions and blankets you need, and as you read the practice through to yourself, let yourself be open to what feels good for you. You might like to prop the book on a cushion, for example, so your arms and hands can relax.

GETTING READY

Welcome to the practice of yoga nidra.

Welcome to this safe, protected place of rest, your true home.

Just arriving here is enough, we've burned the to-do list and the hard part is over.

There is no wrong way to do this.

This is all just an invitation – if there's anything that doesn't sit well with you, you can let it go.

GETTING COMFY

The intention of this practice is to accept the process of Emergence.

Hang up your 'do not disturb' sign, turn off your phone, and create a space to rest, gathering all the cushions and blankets you need to recline comfortably.

Wriggle around to find a position where your shoulders can release a bit more, softly settling back ...

Releasing the jaw with a yawn or a sigh.

Sinking into your resting place.

Letting your eyes soften.

Noticing the sounds beyond the place you are resting in.

Noticing the sounds in the space around you.

Drawing your attention closer to notice the sound of your breath.

THE SEASONS IN THE BREATH

Noticing the breath, the uniqueness of each breath, just soft and effortless.

How each breath holds the Seasonal cycle, each one different and yet the same.

The start of the in-breath is the dawn of Spring,

Coming into the fullness of Summer,

Then releasing into the Autumn of the out-breath,

And the quiet of Winter at the end of the out-breath.

Notice how the Seasons roll effortlessly through the breath, the inevitability of it,

The way your belly rises with the in-breath,

Always follows by the release and emptying of the out-breath;

Spring and Summer bringing you out into the world, and Autumn and Winter bringing you home to yourself …

Name the Seasons of the breath for a few more cycles, with the belly rising and falling. Noticing now the place at the end of the out-breath where it turns into an inhalation, where Spring begins.

There's no need to change anything at all, just notice and enjoy this place of change;

Enjoying the Emergence of the breath for a moment.

INNER SMILE

Take a moment to imagine that something good is coming your way, a pleasing sense of anticipation; good stuff is coming towards you …

Notice how this feels in your body:

Like an inner smile.

KISSING THE BODY AWAKE

Now we're going to take a journey around the body, imagining that each place is being gently kissed awake, by the softest most loving friend …

A soft kiss to the forehead between the eyebrows,

To the jaw, the tongue and throat,

Kisses on the right arm all the way from the shoulder to the palm and a kiss for each fingertip …

Kisses on the left arm, all the way from the shoulder to the palm, and a kiss for each fingertip …

A line of gentle kisses down the centre of the body from the collarbone, over the heart, to the naval, and to the centre of the pubic bone …

Loving kisses all down right leg from the hip, to the knee, the foot and on the tip of each toe.

Loving kisses all down right leg from the hip, to the knee, the foot and on the tip of each toe.

A kiss for the base of the spine, then to each vertebra all the way up to the top of the back, to each shoulder blade …

Kisses for the bones of the neck and the base of the skull

And the softest of kisses to each temple, each eye, the cheeks, tip of the nose and both sides of the jaw,

Feeling the whole body kissed awake by the softest, most loving friend.

PULSATIONS

With every breath in, notice how the kisses call you to awaken, become more alive.

And with every breath out, the kisses soothe you back into yourself.

Breathing in and calling your attention sweetly outwards, breathing out and coming gently back in …

Letting you move effortlessly between these two states of being on the breath.
Follow these pulsations for a few breath cycles.

Now, holding both at the same time, having both the awakening and the sleepy home-coming, both together.
For a moment or two, notice how it is to have both at the same time.

THE INNER JOURNEY OF EMERGENCE

Imagine that you could journey down inside, into the pelvic bowl. Where you find you can rest in a safe, comfortable nest, with just the right kind of softness, just the right cushions and blankets for you to rest perfectly. Look how the gleaming, resilient structure of the pelvis encircles you and holds you safe, free from worries or cares. You are protected here. Take time to admire this beautiful home. Celebrating the resilience of a life lived, and survived. Finding in this safe citadel a place to rest, curling up now in this safe haven, you feel the protection of the pelvic bowl around you, containing you.

And deep in this space there are layers and layers of the sweetest aromatic wrappings, painted with rich reds and golds, with intricate designs and symbols; and woven into the layers are protective herbs with sweet oils. As you enjoy these layers you begin to see there is a potent life force buried here. The layers pull back to reveal a beautiful seed, the shell burnished and pulsating with new life. You see the natural line that marks the two halves of the shell start to deepen and, before your eyes, you witness the miracle of new life emerging from the seed that has rested and waited so long. The life of the tiny, precious seedling starting here, glowing with the light of spring.

You observe that the seedling unfurls herself, emerging according to her own rhythm, shining her light into the area around her, drawing on the resources laid down in the autumn. As you observe the leaves growing, you notice how, when she meets an obstacle, her light will seem to withdraw back into herself for a little time, before she re-orientates herself towards what will nourish her, and grows towards what will sustain her emergence. You find around yourself material that will protect her for her journey ahead, and gifts to nourish her journey, and you store them safely here among the layers of richly coloured wrappings, interweaving the gifts she'll need in the future along with blessings for her journey.

THE SEASONS IN THE BREATH

Noticing the breath once more ...
How each breath holds the Seasonal cycle, each cycle different and yet the same:
The start of the in-breath the dawn of Spring,

Coming into the fullness of Summer,
Then releasing into the Autumn of the out-breath
And the quiet of Winter.
Notice how the Seasons roll effortlessly through you, the inevitability of it,
The way your belly rises with the in-breath,
Always followed by the release and emptying of the out-breath.

INNER SMILE

Take another moment to imagine that something good is coming your way:
A warm openness ready to receive goodness.
Notice how this feels in your body:
Like an inner smile.

RETURNING TO THE HERE AND NOW

Noticing now the sound of your breath,
Expanding your attention to the sounds in the room around you ...
The sounds beyond the room as you come back into the here and now;
Start to expand your awareness of where you are, looking around at your space ...
Start to stretch and move, yawn and wriggle as you come back to the everyday world.

As we close this practice of yoga nidra, explore Emergence and find your own pace.

Wide awake, wide awake and present.
Let yourself move gently from this yoga nidra, giving yourself space before you move back into your everyday life.

Congratulations on giving yourself this rest.

You can find a link to download the audio for this nidra on page 392.

62 Learning to trust

'I TRUST MYSELF AND MY OWN
INSTINCTS ABOUT WHAT I NEED AND
WHO I WANT IN MY LIFE. I TRUST
THOSE WHO HAVE BEEN THROUGH IT
THEMSELVES AND WHO KNOW WHAT
THEY ARE TALKING ABOUT. THOSE
WITH WISDOM OF THE PROCESS.
OTHERWISE THEY ARE TALKING OUT
THEIR BACKSIDE.'

'Tonya'

You're far enough in now. Looking back to your time in Separation, you understand that you can lean into the trust you have developed by knowing you have survived this wild menopause ride. Trust that your body speaks to you as a real and true friend; that you are supported; that when you listen to your inner needs, healing can happen. That the right path will open for you to go forwards, even though you don't quite know where it will lead. Trusting that the right information, people, links, and tools will arrive for you in their own time.

'ALL MY LIFE I HAVE REGARDED TRUST
AS SOMETHING I GIVE OR DON'T GIVE
TO OTHERS. AT THIS STAGE OF MY LIFE
IT HAS BECOME VERY CLEAR THAT THE
MOST IMPORTANT EXPERIENCE OF TRUST
IS ABOUT MYSELF. FOR ME TO BE ABLE TO
LIVE THE LIFE AND BE THE AUTHENTIC
PERSON I WANT TO BE, I HAVE LEARNED
THAT I HAVE TO TRUST. TRUST MYSELF,
TRUST THE PATTERNS AND CYCLES OF LIFE,
MY INNER WORKINGS, AND OF THAT WHICH
WE DON'T UNDERSTAND YET.'

Sharon

You've travelled a long way, baby. Do you remember those first seismic shifts in Separation when you thought that you were going mad? Look how far you've travelled since then and all the kindness and love you have given yourself. Look at how the transformative path has unfolded for you, just by you being present for yourself. All this experience is building up your trust in the process, and helping you understand that pushing yourself and trying to make stuff happen now is not the way forwards. Arriving in Emergence, your capacity to trust becomes extremely useful, because the fresh Spring breeze is just so delicious and the possibility of expanding 'out there' again is tantalizing. As Melanie Santorini, the author of *Majesteria*, explains:

More cooking, more preparation time was still needed ... As time went on, I began to trust the newness of what wanted to emerge through me.[1]

I find this statement reveals the process of Emergence beautifully:

1. It takes its own time to cook.
2. The 'newness' comes from within, rather than being imposed from outside.
3. It comes 'through' us, meaning that for us to act as channels for the work to manifest, we have to get out of our own way! This is the opposite of an ego-led activity; it requires a subtle dance of attention and release.

'THIS HAS BEEN THE BIGGEST PERIOD OF UNCERTAINTY IN MY LIFE AND I'VE MADE SOME MASSIVE CHANGES THAT FELT COMPLETELY MAD AT THE TIME. IT TOOK ME UP SOME FAIRLY MAJOR WRONG TURNS AND MADE ME FACE SOME FAMILY TRUTHS THAT WERE VERY UNCOMFORTABLE. HOWEVER, THERE WAS SO MUCH SYNCHRONICITY DURING THIS PERIOD THAT I ABSOLUTELY TRUSTED IT WAS A PROCESS I HAD TO GO THROUGH, EVEN THOUGH IT WAS BLOODY HORRIBLE AT TIMES.'

Jessica

PRACTICE

- Use the Yoga Nidra for Emergence on pages 317–320 with the intention to trust that your next steps will reveal themselves in their own time.
- Reflect on your menopause journey and see how far you have come since you first noticed signs of being in Separation.
- Explore these prompts with friends, with a daydream or in your journal:
  - What does trust feel like?
  - What do I need in order to trust?

I trust myself and my own instincts, especially when they make no sense.

63 Holding the charge

'Holding the charge' is a powerful technique that comes in especially handy in Emergence; proposed by Red School's menstrual awareness, it's like RAIN on steroids. When we're triggered by something, either internally or externally, our usual response is to move away from the discomfort by reacting through either pushing it away or jumping to an easier option.

Pausing for long enough to hold awareness of both sides of the conflict, and doing nothing, gives us time to cook up a third way – something that can truly serve us. Alexandra Pope and Sjanie Hugo Wurlitzer explain:

> *Instead of reacting to every thought and feeling that floods you at this time, you now have the capacity to 'sit in the stew' and let yourself be cooked. This presence and 'self-holding' is a direct act of love that transforms these reactive and defensive ways into vital elements of your being and becomes the means for you to soften and expand into your Wild Power.* [1]

To soften and expand sounds good, eh? At this point in your process you will have to hold the charge of both longing for and of not knowing your path. Melanie Santorini, author of *Majesteria*, compares it to 'planking' – that core exercise of balancing on toes, elbows, and forearms, which requires us to use our core effectively to spread the load. Likewise, holding the tension requires that we contain our conflict with *as little strain as possible* to ourselves. Holding something *with* tension might look like:

- overthinking
- frantic midnight Googling
- asking everyone's opinion
- blaming and/or picking fights
- throwing everything at once at a problem

Holding something lightly might look like:

- noticing body sensation
- treating yourself with kindness and respect
- trusting the answer will arrive
- naming it when it comes to mind
- finding appropriate support for ourselves from friends, professionals, and circles

PRACTICE

- When you notice you're holding something tightly, extend your out-breath to invite softness into the body.
- Bring your attention to the places where your body is supported, either by your chair or the earth. Amplify the connection by pressing down, stamping or pushing as appropriate.
- Use Tara Brach's RAIN meditation (see chapter 45) to explore the tension you are holding.
- When you are exercising, keep an eye out for how you hold tension in your body and explore how you can soften around it.
- Use your favourite yoga nidra to help you let go.

I am both soft and strong.

64 Learning to receive

'I DID FIND IT HARD TO RECEIVE
AND USED TO THINK IT WAS A SIGN
OF WEAKNESS, BUT I RESENTED THE
FACT THAT OTHERS THOUGHT I DIDN'T
NEED HELP. I DEVELOPED A SHIELD OF:
"I'M OK, I CAN LOOK AFTER MYSELF."
THEN I MOVED BACK IN WITH MY SISTER
AND EXPERIENCED HER NURTURING
GOODNESS AND LET MYSELF HAVE THE
TIME I WANTED TO REST AND BE QUIET
AND REFLECT. I DID WHAT I WANTED TO
DO BY LOOKING AFTER MYSELF. AS AUDRE
LORDE SAID, "WE MUST LEARN TO MOTHER
OURSELVES THEN OUTER RELATIONSHIPS
REFLECT THE INNER SAFETY WE HAVE
CREATED."

Sarah

This is a tough one for us in the early twenty-first century. Can we allow ourselves to be filled with what nourishes us and to really allow ourselves to be as big as we can be? Growing a big, shining light is what menopause is all about, but we have so much conditioning keeping us small and protected, it takes a bit of practice to do this. Girls born into the middle of the twentieth century were trained to put other people first, most especially cis men, and to subsume their own needs – you only have to look at the ongoing pay gap to see it. After a lifetime of giving our energy away to other people and not leaving enough for ourselves, can we change the pattern? Can we not only re-learn how to receive but how to contain and hold on to our energy, rather than give it away?

> ‘I KEPT RUSHING INTO PROJECTS IN EMERGENCE AND THEN FELL ON MY ARSE, NEEDING TO RETREAT RIGHT BACK INTO MY MENOPAUSE CAVE.’
>
> *‘Gil’*

Emergence is a process of moving outward and retreating again, stepping out too far perhaps, then recalibrating and trying a different way. Someone once told me that 99 per cent of the time, the pre-digital aeroplane flew in slightly the wrong direction, needing constant correction from the pilot. We learn by experimenting and finding what is possible, so as we move towards Second Spring, can we allow ourselves to recalibrate, receive goodness and fill ourselves up, without having to give it all away again?

'I SUPPOSE SAYING NO IS ONE WAY
OF ALLOWING MYSELF TO RECEIVE
GOODNESS.'

Kathleen

PRACTICE

Starting small:

Can you let yourself truly absorb a compliment?

- What about your lunch – can you really give it the time needed to prepare and digest it?
- Can you let yourself be heard in your primary relationship?

Then in a bigger sense:

- Can you allow the universe to fill you with awe?
- Can you allow engagement with your delicious girlhood dreams again?

I am open to receive.

65 Finding your calling

It is intimidating to read that we will engage with our calling and give energy to the wider consciousness as Second Springers, especially when we barely have the energy to care for ourselves, let alone those around us. But maybe, just maybe, it's possible that our ovaries have to retire before we can get our direction back from wherever we left it as a teenager.

Let me start this section by stating that I already know what your calling is. Your calling is simply to be more yourself. That's it. That is all you are required to be. And note, that's not 'do' but 'be'. It's not about the big visible project; we might be called to sing in the shower or be amongst the trees. A fabulous guide might be one of my favourite questions: *what would be pleasurable now?* To be a sometime-happy human is *more* than enough. Totally winning. It might be one small thing that calls us, or a dozen different things that might start a steady candle flame. Or a big, public project. We're always drawn to a grand sweep in our stories, yet real life is often more nuanced and subtle.

At primary school, there was a girl in my class called Tabitha who knew what her calling was. She was going to be a show-jumping champion, no question; every moment of her free time was spent dreaming or plotting her progress. Whether she made it or not I don't know, but I always envied her, this knowing what she was about and who she was. My enthusiasms were always a little half-hearted, their uniting thread a desire to be loved and appreciated, never settling on a particular direction.

'MY BODY CLOCK WAS TICKING TO RE-
BIRTH MYSELF, TO DRASTICALLY CHANGE
MY LIFE SITUATION AND RECLAIM MY
FREEDOM. I HAVE NO INTEREST NOW IN
THE "SHOULD" OF LIFE AND FOCUS MORE
ON MY "COULDS", AND I NOW WAKE EACH
DAY WITH MY FOCUS ON MY FULFILLING
MY DREAMS. ALSO, I NOTICE SUCH A FLOW
AND MAGNETISM, WHEN I AM IN FLOW
WITH MY DESIRES AND TRUST IN MYSELF
AND MY ABILITY TO MANIFEST THEM —
GUESS WHAT? — THINGS START HAPPENING
WITHOUT ME TRYING AND OPPORTUNITIES
ARE PRESENTED THAT MATCH THOSE
DESIRES.'

Clare

Looking back over my life I can see how my early experiences of birth and early years set a calling in motion, a karmic lesson to be learned, which in various forms I have shared with the world. I am not alone either. Most healers and therapists I have met get started because they wanted to heal their own wounds and like Chiron, the wounded healer in Greek myth, they then go on to develop expertise that is rooted in their own experience.

If the term 'calling' is too intimidating, suggesting a project that is too BIG and IMPORTANT, then try Caitlin Moran's idea that we simply pursue the things we've always longed to. Each of us, coming through the crucible of menopause armed with tools of discernment, truth-telling, humility, and vulnerability, has something to share with our communities. From my immediate circle, Jane has created a haven for the wildlife in her garden. Leila educates her community about the sacred rites of womanhood. Lorraine has a bloody good time with her grandchildren. Cryn and Alice trained to be yoga teachers and now share their hard-won body wisdom with younger women. Caroline expands her horizons by reading the books she never had time to before.

'MENOPAUSE TAUGHT ME THAT I CAN BE MYSELF. BEFORE, I WAS THE WOMAN WHO NEVER EXPRESSED HERSELF AND HAD TO PLEASE OTHERS AND ALWAYS BOTHERED ABOUT WHAT PEOPLE THOUGHT. I CAN'T BELIEVE HOW HAPPY I AM NOW; POSTMENOPAUSE IT IS THE BEST PART OF MY LIFE.'

Edwina Staniforth, activist and herbalist

And perhaps the greatest calling is that we feel we're able to be ourselves finally. To be able to reclaim more of our shadow, a wider range of being than our lives have allowed so far, and share that with the world.

Calling is not about work or money, but if it provides you with work and earns you a living then you've won twice over. More often, it's about the bit in between, the drifting and pauses, where our attention goes as we spend our days. As the poet Annie Dillard says, how we spend our days is how we spend our lives.[1]

It helps if you come to this with a completely open mind and just follow your nose. Your purpose wants to manifest *through* you so there's no pushing to be done, just a state of mindful attention to cultivate.

PRACTICE

- What are you curious about?
- What feels like fun?
- What fills you up?
- What wound have you healed that you have developed an expertise in?
- Stay open and attentive to the signs and gifts that life brings you.

To be myself is more than enough.

66 Make friends with death

Tick-tock… we are going to die. There, I said it. In fact, we are going to die twice, because our old self is going to die in menopause and be reborn in Second Spring, and then we are going to die at the end of our life. It is time to make friends with death and through this friendship come to appreciate that now is all we've got. We all respond differently when faced with finality of death; some will go slower and smell the roses, some grab their bucket list and get busy with that, some take steps towards forgiveness, some name the perpetrators of their abuse. Whatever the actions taken, it's a movement towards completion. A call to wake up and live as consciously as we possibly can.

The feeling of urgency that our mortality brings can further refine our discernment about what to do with ourselves, and how to live each day as if it were our last. Our newly acute awareness of death makes everything more urgent and fearful – fear of being hurt, fear of loss – but ultimately the way through is by using our awareness to allow the fear. Remember when we went on that bear hunt to feel our feelings in chapter 45? It's the same with the fear of dying: we must 'go through' it to be properly alive.

> 'AS A BUDDHIST, I'VE SPENT SO MANY
> HOURS ON THE CUSHION CONTEMPLATING
> MY OWN DEATH. I HAVE BEEN MENTALLY
> PLANNING THE KIND OF SEND-OFF I'D
> LIKE. THIS MEANS I'D HAVE TO ORGANIZE
> IT NOW TO HEAD OFF ANY PROBLEMS OF
> MY LOVED ONES THROWING A FIT WHEN
> SEEING MY PARTING WISHES.'
>
> *Claire*

We live in a grief-averse culture: death is tidied away quietly and there's praise for moving on from it as quickly as possible. It's changed a little here in the UK after the mass outpouring of grief for Princess Diana in 1997, but generally people do not want to be near our grief because it reminds them of their own losses. Not much room for grieving, but even less to express sadness for the loss of dignity for menopause, the shaming of the menstrual cycle or for the earth. Protect this delicate process from the shaming and blaming of our culture; honour your sadness and grief for what you have lost; give it all the space you need.

'I HAVE TURNED SIXTY AND I KNOW AT ONE LEVEL THAT I AM NEARER TO DEATH. I FIND PART OF THE CHALLENGE IS TAKING STOCK OF THIS KNOWLEDGE WITHOUT DESPAIR AT THE INEVITABILITY OF THE END OF LIFE. I HAVE MADE A WILL AND I THINK FROM TIME TO TIME ABOUT WHAT TYPE OF FUNERAL I WANT.'

'Holly'

The menopause transition is an excellent time to put your affairs in order, to help you release the fear of death and live more lightly. Here are some tasks that will help you release through the fear and ultimately, when the day comes, be very helpful for your nearest and dearest.

PRACTICE

- If you haven't done so already, write your will.
- Talk to your nearest and dearest about what you'd like to happen to your body after you've died.
- Talk about what you'd like to happen if you're incapacitated, and make a living will.
- Think about organ donation and put that in place, telling your next of kin what you want.
- Make an 'in case of emergency' document that includes essential details and explains where to find the following information and documents: birth certificate, your pet's food/ routines, bank, savings and investment details, social media usernames and passwords, website usernames and passwords, national insurance number, contacts for nearest and dearest, property/landlord information.

Emotional Housework

What would you do if you had a year to live? This is the excellent question raised in Stephen Levine's *A Year to Live*, which has meditations and practices you might like to dip into.[1] For a book with reflective musings, check out Zalman Schachter-Shalomi's *From Age-ing to Sage-ing – A Revolutionary Approach to Growing Older.*[2] No make-up tips for 'older skin' here, I'm afraid; instead you'll find a lot of great exercises for gaining forgiveness and closure in your life. Here are some actions you might consider to help clear the emotional baggage:

- Let go of possessions; Marie Kondo is your friend.
- Write a letter to yourself from your deathbed.
- Who do you need to forgive? You could write a letter to them and send or burn it.
- Which relationships do you need to let go of?
- Use the Clearing Meditation (see pages 54–56), if that speaks to you.
- Reflect methodically on each decade of your life, allowing yourself to name your challenges with compassion, and celebrate yourself.

Everything goes away, eventually.

67 Redefine how to be a woman

We learn how to be women from our mothers or female caregivers. As we grow up, we view these lessons with a critical eye and perhaps learn instead how to be the person our mother was not. Our culture tells us how to be women through magazines, movies, and social media – and even though we know it's airbrushed and unrealistic, somehow, like gas seeping under the door, we can't help but breathe it in. The poisonous gas of patriarchy fills us with unease that our bodies are not up to scratch, that we should be working harder, more successful, kinder, sexier, the 'right' skin colour, more 'feminine', more, more … Often we can't identify why we are insufficient and bathe in a general sense of lacking somehow.

'SOMETIMES I LOOK DISPARAGINGLY AT MY WRINKLY HANDS AND FACE. HOWEVER, OVERALL, I FEEL MORE CONFIDENT AND HAPPIER WITH MY APPEARANCE NOW THAN I EVER DID AS A YOUNGER WOMAN. I REFUSE TO USE ANY OF THE ANTI-AGEING PRODUCTS THAT OUR CULTURE THROWS AT US. IF I FEEL MYSELF GETTING CRITICAL, I KNOW THAT I AM INTERNALIZING SOCIETY'S PREJUDICE AND I PRACTISE LOVING MYSELF FOR WHO I AM.'

'Caroline'

As our outmoded identities crack and fall away, and we've healed some more chunks of our life, menopause gives us the chance to push aside what we've learned from our families and culture, and think about what kind of person we would like to be now. As the founder of the True Style Journey e-courses, Leesa Whisker, explained to me, it can be an opportunity to reimage ourselves from the outside in:

Style-wise, perimenopause is a potent time of reinvention. It's a time of untethering from external notions of how a woman should look and be to start dressing as you damn please, creating a style that feels as good as it looks. It's a joyous and liberating journey that can transform more than just your wardrobe.

Emergence gives us a chance to remove ourselves from the gas-filled house and step out of binary restrictions to ask, 'Who am I now?' A friend talked to me about the need to pause and consider where she is, to 'update herself'; at this phase of Emergence she's evolving so fast she can't keep up with herself.

'I'VE HELD THE VERY OUTDATED VIEW THAT FEMININITY WAS A FLOATY-SKIRT-WEARING, DELICATE AND GRACEFUL WOMAN WHO DIDN'T MAKE A FUSS AND LIKED MAKING CAKES AND BEING NICE TO PEOPLE. I'VE JUST REALIZED THAT THIS IMAGE IS STILL IN MY UNCONSCIOUS AND THEREFORE I'VE NEVER IDENTIFIED MYSELF AS FEMININE. GOOD GRIEF, NO WONDER! SO ACTUALLY, FEMININITY IS: NURTURER, BEING ABLE TO BE VULNERABLE (WHICH IS INCREDIBLY STRONG), RECEIVER, POWERFUL, LIFE GIVER, INTUITIVE, CREATIVE, COMMUNICATOR, NETWORKER, SUPPORTER, LOVER.'

Sandra

In long-term relationships, the redefining process often shows up as a problem. When menopause has forcibly propelled us into growth, maybe our partner has stayed static, or alternatively perhaps both partners have grown in opposite directions. It's mostly women in transition (in transit!) who initiate divorce, with men being caught off-guard.[1] Author Darcey Steinke came up with the delightful term 'gender slippage'[2], and the notion of the 'late blooming lesbian' or as a friend calls it a 'Gonegay' is not only for privileged celebrities, it's a statistical reality.[3, 4]

Over on the gender front, young people often feel much more empowered today to choose a different way of identifying themselves, so why shouldn't menopause perform the same refinement at the other end of our reproductive life? After all, we've had another thirty years of lived experience to explore what it all means and to choose again an identity that better fits our souls. Perhaps we could take on the 'stridently mannish' stance that the eighteenth-century medics despised, and own it in as part of the 21st-century's gender-fluid liberation? The decline in oestrogen is not a universally negative experience; perhaps we can feel more the balance of the masculine within us, especially once our hormones come into steadiness in Second Spring and our testosterone levels are healthy. Menopause: the great balancer! This is not a story that is often told.

'DON'T BE SURPRISED IF YOU QUESTION YOUR GENDER AT MENOPAUSE.'

Samantha

If you are content with your sexual and gender identity, then what does that mean? It can be hard to see beyond the confines of what we have been taught, but menopause with its internal focus gives us excellent tools and the time to unravel the tangled strings of who we are in terms of our womanhood. This is where Inner-Season awareness is particularly helpful, because it draws our attention to all aspects of our being, allowing us to trace the strings as they emerge. To the Spring qualities of delight, newness and wobbliness, the Summer of being 'out there', exposure and showing ourselves, the Autumn of rage, grief, truth-telling, discernment and the Winter of deep self-knowing and spirituality. And everything in between. It gives us both our power and our loss, our exposure and our quietness. The process of menopause can serve to integrate all of this so we can own more of ourselves.

'I FEEL THAT NO FEAR, GRAB EVERY EXPERIENCE AND LIVE EVERY MOMENT FEELING. I'M BACK! THIS IS THE "ME" FROM BEFORE.'

Clare

PRACTICE

Use these prompts for writing or as a jumping off point for a conversation:

- What does it mean to you, to be a woman? What are the positives and negatives?
- What meaning does femininity hold for you? What can you welcome and what do you wish to leave behind?
- Use the Womb Journey Meditation (see pages 147–148) to explore your inner landscape.

Who shall I be today?

68 We need role models

There was a particular moment when I was entering Separation that older women started to catch my eye. I remember listening to childbirth educator Penny Simkin[1] give a talk and being blown away not so much by the content (which was excellent) but by how *she* was. At this time, she must have been in her Second Summer, and I loved the power of her authority built from enabling thousands of abuse survivors to give birth safely. She radiated humour and humility about herself and her achievements. She wore her power lightly – in a way I had not seen in men of a similar age. This combination of authority and humility totally does it for me.

If you fancy a literary role model, how about the French author Colette, whose Second Spring brought a terrific burst of energy: writing, touring plays, new lovers, travelling? At the age of 59, on the cusp of her Second Summer, she opened a beauty shop in Paris, just for fun. Needless to say, everyone flocked to receive a facial from the great writer. If Colette's facials are too fanciful, then what about Kristin Scott Thomas's character in the TV series *Fleabag*? She shows up in a bar and gently turns down Fleabag's advances, while saying how she's feeling free and no longer 'a machine with parts'. Screenwriter Phoebe Waller-Bridge gives her the awesome line:

I've given birth to a darling bundle of self-esteem.[2]

And who doesn't long for that? Once we've given birth to our darling bundle of self-esteem, it requires tending and nurturing through our Second Spring so that, like Penny Simkin, we can stand up for what we believe in and make a difference in the world. Or take scholar and activist Lydia Ruyle, who at 60 started a project to make *The Goddess Banners*, 300 visionary images of the Sacred Feminine drawn from all cultures, which travelled the world from Machu Picchu to Glastonbury. The biopic of her life *Herstory*[3] is well worth watching, most especially for her joyful attitude to death.

I am very lucky in that I have two awesome Second Spring role models in my sisters. I'm the youngest sibling by seven years, so at every point in my life, I have witnessed them being their unique version of tender, strong, and singing their truth. But in the everyday world, how many older women do you actually see looking comfortable in their authority? On the TV, the newsreaders all look under forty, no matter what their real age, and the wage gap in the entertainment industry is grossly unequal. If there were more older women visible in leadership roles, who were able to carry both their authority *and* their vulnerability, we would know that menopause isn't the end of life and that nourishing our tenderness opens the door to connection and change.

For an example of inspiring fictional role models, there is the witch Serafina Pekkala in Philip Pullman's novels who at around 300 years old, holds her power with magnificence and the bearing of a panther. When your inner-panther is feeling a bit wobbly, leopard print should never underrated as an instant fix.

Next up, I'd like to introduce you to Viv Albertine. Unless you're a fan of punk music you may have missed her, so I'll say a little about her life. She exploded onto the punk scene as part of *The Slits*, an all-girl band who exemplified the DIY ethos of punk and revolutionized how women were able to create in the music world. What makes me a total fan is her memoir Clothes, Clothes, Clothes. Music, Music, Music. Boys, Boys, Boys. Friends with the Sex Pistols and The Clash, she was always an outsider, and writes with an honesty that is absolutely moving about struggling with body image, surviving cancer, marriage, dating, loneliness, and the nitty-gritty of life we all experience. Viv Albertine's memoir follows her re-entry into the world. Having ended her marriage, she surfs the creative wave of Emergence and starts making anonymous appearances at open-mike gigs. Though her skills seem to have deserted her, she feels the compulsion to get the songs out there, they need to be heard.

I love this description of Emergence: the way her creative energy has a path of its own and all Viv has to do is channel it in a way that is manageable for her; it is emerging through her. To jump onto YouTube or a London stage would be too much too soon. She soothes her vulnerability by finding a safe way of allowing it expression. And when the blokes in the random pub chat through her set, she calls them out.[5]

Sometimes you pick on the wrong middle-aged woman. Fast forward to 2009 and her song 'Confessions of a MILF' is an utterly joyous celebration of her transition from domesticated female in Separation to Second Spring creative. Search it out on YouTube and let yourself sink into the chorus listing the activities she has left behind her:

'cooking, cleaning, baking, washing, faking, fucking, cleaning, shopping'[6]

This is emphatically not trying to recapture her youthful role of punk innovator (or filmmaker or wife or writer) but following the flow of her creativity. Her direct gaze, searing honesty, and stylish clothes do not speak of hiding. After her middle years of being an outsider with no space allowed for her to create, she can take her space; vulnerable, funny and absolutely present. Like I said, I am a fan.

Also on my list are academic Mary Beard, poet and musician Patti Smith, actor Meryl Streep, media tycoon Oprah, author and civil rights activist Maya Angelou, and designer and activist Vivienne Westwood. Clearly in the arts and creative world, there is more room for self-expression and living beyond a conventional role. The common denominator? Apart from their visibility, it's that they're all slightly scary and have an absolute commitment to following their truth.

'BE PREPARED TO DO OUTRAGEOUS THINGS.'

'Jas'

PRACTICE

- Practise the Yoga Nidra for Emergence (see pages 317–320).
- Make a list of the older women you admire.
- What qualities do you love about them?
- How can you identify and nourish these qualities in yourself?

Give no fucks.

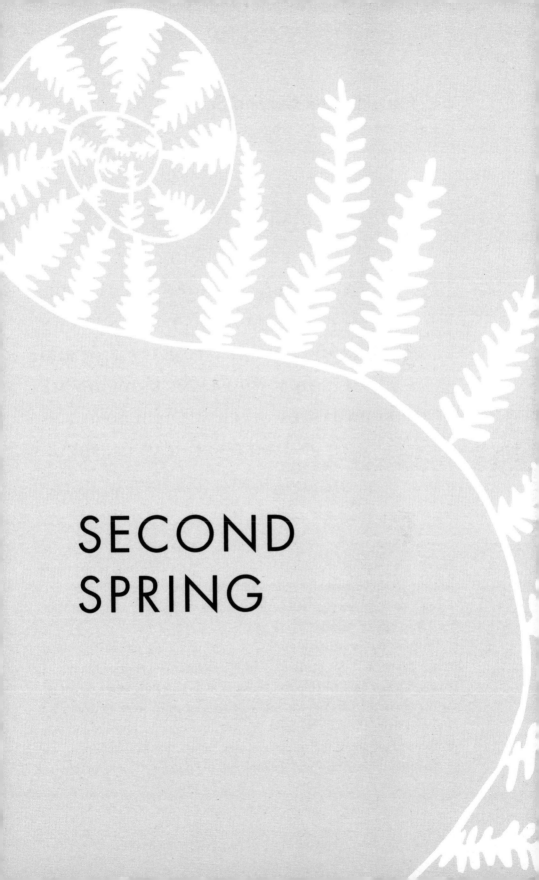

SECOND
SPRING

69 You will enter Second Spring

'THERE'S A BRAZENNESS ABOUT IT. THERE ARE MULTIPLE LAYERS BECAUSE I AM MORE VULNERABLE AS I AGE, BUT IT'S SUCH AN INCREDIBLE RELIEF TO HAVE FIGURED OUT WHO I AM. KNOWING MY BOUNDARIES GIVES ME FREEDOM; IT'S LIKE BEING UNLEASHED.'

Alexandra Pope, co-founder of Red School

There is a raucous crowd of Second Springers cheering you on and sending you love across the ether. And from the wild seas of Separation, if you look through your telescope, you can see them as a light on your horizon, a city of angels.

Imagine the best party-guest list ever, including Michelle Obama fresh from her sell-out world tour for her memoir *Becoming* or Madonna, having ditched Guy Ritchie and become the best-selling single artist of the decade in the US. You can see what these women were up to as they emerged from their menopause process into Second Spring, and you probably know about the amazing achievements that followed.

Yes, they have status and wealth, and in Madonna's case a team of people to do her self-care for her. Personally, I'm not a great fan of celebrity culture. But. They can show us the public face of what happens when we value ourselves in Second Spring and beyond.

'MENOPAUSE IS A RITE OF PASSAGE; IT TAKES WOMEN THROUGH TO EMBODY OUR WISE WOMAN. I WAS MEDITATING A LOT, AND GOING INSIDE MYSELF, A NECESSARY PART OF THE PASSAGE. I CAME THROUGH THAT INTO A MUCH DEEPER PLACE.'

Lynne Franks

Many famous women don't speak publicly about their menopause – which would be career-suicide in the youth-obsessed entertainment industry – but browsing Wikipedia, you'll see the signs: illness, accidents, 'a quiet period in her career', divorce, breakdown, losing friends, mental illness followed by new directions, new relationships, clarity, new projects, and successes.

If I think about the Second Spring people in my life, it's their eyes that speak most clearly to me – sparkling with mischief, engagement, delight in the world. I saw many of them at the Extinction Rebellion gatherings; I would catch their eye and a massive, connected beam of a smile would follow. These are not people who are 'settling' for what life has given them; they are carving out the future for themselves and their communities.

'IT'S A PROCESS ABOUT FINDING WHO I REALLY, REALLY AM, WHAT MY VOICE SHOULD BE, HOW SHOULD I SPEAK MY TRUTH, WHAT IS MY TRUTH, HOW DO I CONNECT TO THE EARTH WITH MY FEET. THEY'RE INDICATIVE OF A PERSON WHO FEELS (IN A SQUEAKY VOICE) – "OH, I'M NOT SURE I WANT TO BE HERE, I'M NOT STANDING, I CAN'T STAND, I CAN'T ACCEPT THIS EXPERIENCE" – TO UNRAVEL ALL THAT IS A LONG PROCESS. MY FEET ARE UNBELIEVABLY DIFFERENT FROM WHEN I STARTED AGED 50, REALLY DIFFERENT. AND SO AM I.'

Cryn

Personal is political. The changes we make in our Second Spring are not just about us, they are part of a growing movement. There have never been so many educated, enlightened people reaching menopause and asking, 'What's next?' What we choose makes a difference to the broad political life of our world.

Studies have shown that at ovulation, women have evolved to be more competitive for high-status sexual partners and promotion.[1] Known as 'intra-sexual competition', it's also been shown to be cloaked by 'friendliness' to create alliances that disarm potential rivals. In Second Spring, when the ability to reproduce is no longer present, does the competition dissolve along with the oestrogen high? No prizes for guessing that I couldn't find any research, but I would suggest that the impulse in Second Springers to work together for the good of the community is a huge benefit of lower oestrogen. Now that is something you seldom hear, so I'll say it again: a huge benefit of lower oestrogen. Plus, according to the research, at ovulation we have 'an attentional bias toward ornamental objects',[2] so in Second Spring we'll spend less money on all the adornment required to outmanoeuvre our rivals every month. Win–win.

Over the years we have had lots of experience of bumping up against glass ceilings, of calling people out, of #metoo, of being underestimated and ignored, but now with the added testosterone of Second Spring, we have the daring to step beyond what may have limited us in our earlier life. As broadcaster Kirsty Wark put it in the BBC documentary *Menopause and Me*:

Once you've been through it, you go, 'That's it, I can do anything now!'[3]

Where we chose to put our money, whether savings or spending, makes a difference. You wouldn't think we existed at all if you look at ads on the television; indeed, to find any convincing images of women in Second Spring is unusual. But we have the power to support businesses whose ethics we admire and withdraw our spending from those we do not.

How do I know if I'm in Second Spring?

The cross-over from Winter into Spring is a tender one. We emerge like a newborn calf with wobbly legs, unused to the bright lights – but how do you know when you're finally there? Many of us can only view our arrival in retrospect; it certainly doesn't have much to do with the tidy medical model of a year since your last bleed. It's perfectly possible to have another period more than a year later (though to be on the safe side, it's good to check with your doctor, as postmenopausal bleeds can be an indication of endometrial cancer).

I tried to keep track of the number of days and the weird un-bleed-bleeds that I had, with nine to fourteen-month intervals, to see if I was 'there' yet. But in the end, I gave up, decided it was irrelevant, and that I was where I was – and that, ironically, was probably the point at which I landed in Second Spring. I could tell I was there because I no longer cared where I was.

There are many ways I could describe it. I had the sense of having landed somewhere or having arrived in a different internal landscape. It was defined for me also as a negative, by the *absence* of change. I no longer felt the great, swirling undertow of the menopause process swooshing me about. I had landed and found myself in unknown territory. As I still had no clue about it, I asked my wise colleague Leora, who said:

> *I saw in Kate an unfurling. Your focus seemed to gradually shift from the entirety of the inward-looking process, which sometimes appeared painful, to the way you began emerging into the outside world. You shared your work and ideas the world with a new lightness. There also seemed a lightening in the need to be contained and be more carefree, a lightness of giving less fucks.*

Less fucks: that about covers it. You might start to fill your diary up again, to reach out for more social contact. You might be ready to start a new project or resume an old one in a different way. You might find yourself playing with different identities as you try on different hats for size, real and metaphorical, to see which you fancy wearing today. But wearing them lightly now, enjoyed for their beauty and discarded once their time is passed.

'FOR ME IT WAS A LIGHTENING FEELING. I FELT CALMER AND CLEARER. I COULD FEEL MY SWITCHING OFF AND MY PERIODS GOT LIGHTER. USUALLY BEFORE MY BLEED I WOULDN'T BE ABLE TO PARK THE CAR BUT ONE DAY I COULD! SO, FOR ME IT HAS BEEN A TIME OF CLARITY AND TUNING IN ON A DEEPER LEVEL. AND NOW IN MY LATE FIFTIES, I FEEL I AM MORE IN TUNE THAN EVER WITH MYSELF AND ALSO MORE ACCEPTING OF MY DIFFERENT MOODS WHICH FEEL LESS INTENSE. I FEEL THAT I CAN BE WHO I AM.'

Suzanne Yates, founder of Wellmother

In *Crones Don't Whine*, a 125-page hymn of praise to Second Spring, author and Jungian analyst Jean Shinoda Bolen says Second Spring is all about inner development, of being truly oneself, allowing expressions and action with wisdom and ease.

Maybe there are themes from your teenage years arising, the same passions and interests, now presenting themselves with the appreciation won from the understanding that they are gifts, not a given.

Teenager again

Psychiatrist Elisabeth Kübler-Ross, whose work on death and dying inspired the hospice movement, called adolescence – our first Spring – 'the birth of the soul'. Second Spring can be seen as the *rebirth* of the soul, the potent start of a whole new trip round the cycle.

We can expect themes from our adolescence to show up here too. At 13, we had to learn about the constrictions of growing up and the boundaries that held and/or restricted us. Here in Second Spring, we're not worrying about what others think, and we have self-confidence born of a life of finding our way round glass ceilings. We can now locate our own boundaries for ourselves. By consciously calling in our teenager to our Second Spring, we can access more of her lust for life.

'I HONESTLY HAVE ACCESS TO MYSELF
IN A WAY I HAVEN'T FOR YEARS.'

Juliet

Learning where our new boundaries are in the familiar/unfamiliar territory of Second Spring can be painful. For example, now the Second Spring sunshine warms me up, I constantly over-do it with social contact, with work projects, with too much people-time … and then I crash and burn in a frazzled heap. It's a common misconception that once menopause is over we will 'go back to how we used to be before', but this is not the case.

We have undergone an initiation and are fundamentally changed by it. We are also older, and ageing brings constrictions with it, depending on your genetic inheritance and how you have 'spent' your life.

Second Spring brings with it a great creative burst, more energy, and unfettered by expectations, extraordinary things can happen. Check out Georgia O'Keeffe, who settled in New Mexico at the age of 62 and created some of her most evocative work. Welcome to the army of Second Spring folk, standing in our truth.

PRACTICE
- Use the Yoga Nidra for Second Spring (see pages 356–359).

Each Winter is followed by a uniquely precious Spring.

Yoga Nidra for Second Spring

This nidra will give you about 15 minutes of deep rest. Find a cosy space where you can recline undisturbed, with all the cushions and blankets you need, and as you read the practice through to yourself, let yourself be open to what feels good for you. You might like to prop the book on a cushion, for example, so your arms and hands can relax ...

GETTING READY

Welcome to the practice of yoga nidra.

Welcome to this safe, protected place of rest, to your true home.

Just arriving here is enough, we've burned the to-do list and the hard part is over.

There is no wrong way to do this.

This is all just an invitation – if there's anything that doesn't sit well with you, you can let it go.

GETTING COMFY

The intention of this practice is to accept the process of Second Spring.

Hang up your 'do not disturb' sign, turn off your phone, and create a space to rest, gathering all the cushions and blankets you need to recline comfortably.

Wriggle around to find a position where your shoulders can release a bit more, softly settling back ...

Releasing the jaw with a yawn or a sigh.

Sinking into your resting place.

Letting your eyes soften.

Noticing the sounds beyond the place you are resting in.

Noticing the sounds in the space around you.

Drawing your attention closer to notice the sound of your breath.

THE SEASONS IN THE BREATH

Name the Seasons of the breath for a few more cycles with the belly rising and falling.

Noticing now the place at the beginning of the in-breath, the beginning of Spring.

There's no need to change anything at all, just notice and enjoy this place of change.

Enjoying the Spring of the breath for a moment or two.

INNER SMILE

Take a moment to imagine that something good is coming your way, a pleasing sense of anticipation; good stuff is coming towards you ...

Notice how this feels in your body:

Like an inner smile.

SPRING SUN SHINING ON THE BODY

You're going to take a journey, visiting places in the body and imagining the warmth of
the spring sun shining ...

Warm sunshine on the forehead between the eyebrows,

Shining down onto the jaw, the tongue and throat,

A wash of warm sun travelling down the right arm from the shoulder to each fingertip,

A wash of warm sun travelling down the left arm from the shoulder to each fingertip,

A sunbeam tracking and warming the torso from collar bone, through the heart, the navel,
and down to the pubic bone,

A wash of sunshine travelling down the right leg from the hip to the tip of each toe,

A wash of sunshine travelling down the left leg from the hip to the tip of each toe,

Sunshine on your bum,

Then the base of the spine upwards is washed by a wave of sunshine all up the back ...

Sun shining on the back of the neck,

Washing over the crown of the head,

The sun warming the temples, the eyes, cheeks, nose and jaw ...

The whole body full of sunshine ...

The whole body.

PULSATIONS

With every breath in, notice how the sunshine seems to expand to fill the whole body
with warmth and vitality.

And with every breath out, the warmth contracts and concentrates into your pelvis.

Breathing in and filling the whole body, breathing out and focusing on the intense warmth
in the pelvis;

Letting you move effortlessly between these two states of being on the breath,

The light spreading out on the in-breath and bringing it deep inside you on the out-breath.

Follow these pulsations for a few breath cycles,

Now holding both at the same time, having both the whole-body vitality and the intense
warmth in the pelvis, both together;

For a moment or two notice how it is to have both at the same time.

INNER JOURNEY OF SECOND SPRING

Imagine that you could journey down inside, into the pelvic bowl. Where you find you can
rest in a safe, comfortable nest, with just the right kind of softness, just the right cushions
and blankets for you to rest perfectly. Look how the gleaming, resilient structure of the
pelvis encircles you and holds you safe, free from worries or cares. You are protected
here. Take time to admire this beautiful home. Celebrating the resilience of a life lived,
and survived. Finding in this safe citadel a place to rest, curling up now in this safe haven,
you feel the protection of the pelvic bowl around you, containing you.

You see before you a young tree, a sapling, her new leaves gleaming in the spring sunshine. Bright green and just at the moment of unfurling. You can rub your fingers across the leaves and feel their texture; you smell the scent of wet earth, left by the recent rain. And you become aware of the sound of other young trees, all around you, a whole grove of beautiful trees, each one unique in their stance and colouring ... You hear the sound of many leaves shaking and trembling in the warm spring breeze.

Looking down, you see that there are tools left for you to provide the nourishment and safety that this beautiful tree needs to flourish. There is protection to shield her from the hungry woodland creatures; there is support for her to keep her anchored when the spring storms blow in; there is a container with the particular nourishment she needs for her roots and for her foliage. Take some time now to use the tools and equipment around you to protect, support, and nourish your sapling. You find you know exactly what is needed and it comes easily to you to tend to this beautiful tree so that she can establish herself in this new place. When your tasks are completed, your attention is drawn again to the sweet sound of her leaves rustling in the breeze and you catch the words she has for you. Sending her blessings now in words and gifts before you depart.

THE SEASONS IN THE BREATH

Noticing the breath once more ...
How each breath holds the Seasonal cycle, each cycle different and yet the same:
The start of the in-breath the dawn of Spring,
Coming into the fullness of Summer,
Then releasing into the Autumn of the out-breath
And the quiet of Winter.
Notice how the Seasons roll effortlessly through you, the inevitability of it,
The way your belly rises with the in-breath,
Always followed by the release and emptying of the out-breath.

INNER SMILE

Take another moment to imagine that something good is coming your way:
A warm openness ready to receive goodness.
Notice how this feels in your body:
Like an inner smile.

RETURNING TO THE HERE AND NOW

Noticing now the sound of your breath,

Expanding your attention to the sounds in the room around you ...

The sounds beyond the room as you come back into the here and now;

Start to expand your awareness of where you are, looking around at your space ...

Start to stretch and move, yawn and wriggle as you come back to the everyday world.

As we close this practice of yoga nidra, explore Second Spring and find your own pace.

Wide awake, wide awake and present.

Let yourself move gently from this yoga nidra, giving yourself space before you move back into your everyday life.

Congratulations on giving yourself this time to rest.

You can find a link to download the audio for this nidra on page 392.

70 Caring for your Second Spring self

Even if you have allowed the menopause process to hold you through your transformation and been able to tend sweetly to yourself, Second Spring can be a bit of a shock. If you're deep in the trials of Separation when you read this, you probably won't believe me, but the light, after so much winter darkness, can be blinding and it can be a vulnerable process as we emerge. Picture our butterfly ready to emerge from its chrysalis: its wings are not yet ready to be used; in fact, they're still small, wilted, and wrinkled, and immediately need body fluids pumped into their wing veins to develop them. When the wings are plumped up to full size, the butterfly must rest for several hours to let its body dry and harden before flying for the first time.

'I'M GENERALLY FEELING MORE EMPOWERED AND "ON IT" THAN AT ANY OTHER TIME IN MY LIFE, BUT THERE ARE MOMENTS WHEN I CAN'T ARTICULATE WHAT I AM EVEN THINKING, LET ALONE WHAT I'M TRYING TO SAY. TAKING A FEW DEEP BREATHS, AND REMINDING MYSELF TO BE KIND TO MYSELF, OFTEN GIVES ME A DIFFERENT PERSPECTIVE. YESTERDAY, I WAS XENA WARRIOR PRINCESS AND, TODAY, I AM CHANNELLING BAGPUSS.'

Fern

In psychological terms, there's a time in early Second Spring where we are letting our new 'self' harden and dry out from the storms of the menopause process. One of the pitfalls here is that now we're not in menopause, we feel we have to know what we're about, have a plan, get shit done. We feel all the urgency of life and the rush of new energy, but can't yet find our path and it can feel like we've blown it. This is where the hard lessons learned in Emergence are really tested, our capacity to be patient, to hold our energy and trust the process of life.

Second Spring is, well, Spring! Remember those qualities of your first Spring in your teens? The wandering around aimlessly, getting distracted, falling in love, falling into despair, of finding a thousand ways to look outward to find an enticing looking path ... This is a time of new energy, yes, but a time of discovery, because Second Summer is yet to come. It is in Second Summer that the energy moves us once again towards manifesting 'out there' in the world.

In my practice with menstruating clients, I often see how difficulties in their Summer have been triggered by rushing out of their menstrua-tion too quickly into Spring. Having rested and slowed down in their Winter, the pressure to get back out there again can be so strong that there is no time to plump their wings before getting stuck into life; and then exhaustion and fatigue shows up in their Summer. The Life Seasons are no different: shooting out of the Winter of menopause like a cannonball is not going to make for a satisfying Second Summer. One of the primary self-care practices of Second Spring is to take your time, smell the roses, and take deep pleasure in mere existence and the awesome world we live in.

'POSTMENOPAUSE, I FEEL MORE AT HOME INSIDE AND OUT THAN I HAVE EVER FELT ... I HAVE FOUND MY TRIBE OF WONDERFUL WOMEN WHO I'VE BEEN SEARCHING FOR ALL MY LIFE. I LOVE MY WORK, I ENJOY MY LIFE, AND I'M FINDING NEW LOVE AGAIN. I FEEL HOPE THAT THIS IS THE BLOSSOMING OF A NEW BEGINNING OF LIFE THAT SURELY DOES COME THROUGH DEATH, THE ULTIMATE CHANGE AND TRANSFORMATION. IF I'M RIGHT, AS I'M TOLD, THAT THE BEST IS YET TO COME THEN: *WOOOHEY*! BRING IT ON. THE SIXTIES ARE GREAT!'

Liza

One of the kind people who agreed to share her story with me, when she saw I had written about Second Spring, said, 'Oh no, not more happy-clappy bollocks.' It is not my intention to gloss over the reality of ageing and the absolute need to care *even more* lovingly for an older body. We're never the finished article and there's always work to do, inside and out. I truly hope that by now, through the school room of menopause, your self-care is non-negotiable to the point it's not even noticeable as 'self-care' any more, it's just what you do.

'I HAVE LEARNED TO BE KINDER TO
MYSELF, TO OPEN DOORS AND RUN
BATHS, APPLY MOISTURISER AND REST
IN BED OR ON THE SOFA SWATHED
IN BLANKETS. I'VE LEARNED TO
TREAT MYSELF LIKE A DEAR AND
TRUSTED FRIEND.'

Melanie

Food, movement, friendships, creativity, spirituality, sensuality, nature, fun ... all these things have to be an ongoing, nourishing part of our commitment to ourselves if we are to live a satisfying life into our Second Summer, Autumn and Winter.

Self-love is non-negotiable now.

71 You need a party

Arriving at the beginning of a whole new cycle is a potent time. You have been fully worked by the process of menopause. It has tenderized you, cracked you open, sent you deep inside to find your truth – *and you survived!* Despite not being mentored, despite your culture telling you that you were mad, despite being shamed, despite being sold a thousand lies to keep you powerless and obedient to cultural norms, you survived and THRIVED!

Welcome to the next part of your life!

This achievement needs celebrating. The commitment to yourself and to your truth needs to be witnessed and appreciated so you can integrate the full wonder that you are: perfect, whole, and complete. How would you like to do that? How can you witness the wonder that is you and say, "Yes, I am perfect as I am, no fixing required"?

'I WAS HONOURED FOR MY WORK IN WOMEN'S HEALTH AND AS A MOTHER AT MY MENOPAUSE CEREMONY. WITNESSED BY THIRTY WOMEN, INCLUDING MY TEENAGE DAUGHTER AND HER FRIEND. I WAS GUIDED TO THE CENTRE OF THE CIRCLE AND ASTOUNDED BY A FIRE DANCER WHO BLESSED US ALL WITH HER CEREMONIAL DANCE. EVER SINCE, MY CREATIVITY HAS UNBOUNDED RESOURCES AND EXPRESSION AND I FEEL LIKE A WOMAN OF STRENGTH, WISDOM, AND UNIVERSAL LOVE.'

Kayler Becker, reproductive health educator

For some it's a ceremony. For some it's tea at the Ritz or cocktails or dinner. Some of us want it to be a private reflection; others thrive in the reflection of their friends' love. However, you do it, acknowledging this rite of passage is life-changing and if you feel you've missed out, like your menarche, it's never too late to celebrate and mark the transition.

'IT'S ABOUT STANDING IN OUR SOVEREIGNTY, IN THE FULLNESS OF WHO WE ARE. NOW'S THE TIME.'

Bryn Truett-Chavez, menopause mentor and cheerleader

PRACTICE

- Think about how you would like to celebrate your transition: ceremonies can include a ritualized physical walk from one place to the next, a Croning ceremony, songs and poetry – the only limit is your imagination.
- Take some time to write or tell someone the story of your menopause transition: who you were before, who you are now, and what you hope to be.
- You might like to find a way to record your story, in images, words, audio, or film so that you can inspire and educate the women coming after you.
- You could buy or make yourself a piece of jewellery, a garment or object that reflects your Second Spring self.

You are the Empress of your world.

72 Welcome home to yourself

The party poppers are littering the floor and the empty glasses are sticking to the tables. We are done here. You've arrived in a peculiar place of non-movement after all the upheaval you've been through. Time to take a breath.

Congratulations, you have earned your place in Second Spring. Are you completely healed? Of course not. Do you know exactly what is going on? Nope. Are you more comfortable in your skin now? Almost certainly. Are you a beautiful, wise, vulnerable, strong, empowered queen who gives no fucks? Hell, yes!

Whether you've just dipped into the bits that seem relevant to you or read through the whole book, chapter by chapter, thank you for sticking with me. I hope that my words have given you some comfort and that you've picked up a useful thing or two. It's time for me to say goodbye for now, but I can't wait to hear about your adventures in menopause.

Keep talking about your experiences with your friends, work colleagues, and family: together we can change the way our transitions are perceived. Every story that we share creates a little ripple and somewhere, someone feels less alone in their experience. A third of the world are in menopause and postmenopause right now; what shall we create together?

When in doubt, be gentle with yourself and give no fucks.

Acknowledgements

I always had a lot of words, just not necessarily in the right order. The ordering of these words would never have been possible without the help of a great many people – it turns out it takes a whole village to raise a book. The ideas that were ignited by the beautiful hearts and brains of Sjanie and Alexandra at Red School had life breathed into them by the clients and retreat participants that I have been lucky enough to encounter. The content of these pages is built from their courage, generosity and trust. Nothing would have happened at all without the many conversations, ponderings and Circles I have held with Leora Leboff, my dear friend and partner in kindness at Woman Kind. I have been very lucky in receiving ongoing cheerleading, encouragement, and scooping up off the floor from my dear writerly friends Kim Davies and Claire Murphy. Claire has opened up innumerable opportunities for me to explore consciousness, poetry, and writing in her classes, which have greatly contributed to the content here. Juliet Cox, Kelly Holmes, Leora Leboff, Lottie Randomly, and Lisa de Jong were kind enough to read my words and use their sharp, compassionate minds to offer improvements. Hilary Lewin has been a generous traveller in the road to getting this published, sharing the journey and also kindly introducing me to book-doula Celina Wilde. I have so much gratitude to Milli Hill, who kindly introduced me to my agent, Jane Graham Maw. The kindness and help I have received from the team at HarperCollins has been a gift, thank you all for believing in me. Never mind the book, I probably wouldn't be able to function *at all* without the holding from my awesome peers: Barbara Hussong, Liza Waller, Sara Macgregor, Caroline Duggan, Abi Denyer-Bewick, and Lisa de Jong. And the awesome Fuckettes, I bloody love you lot. Finally, my dear partner Ian has held me and everything else together while I've been in menopause-land. You are an utter champion.

Notes

INTRODUCTION

1. Margaret Mead, interviewed by David Frost on *The David Frost Show*, episode #2 (19 Feb. 1970).

2. The psychological phases of Separation, Surrender and Emergence were first identified in the phases of menstruation by Lara Owen. Red School further developed the idea into 'The Five Chambers of Menstruation' and identified them in menopause too. At Woman Kind, Leora Leboff and I realigned the phases and Seasons to match our and our clients' experiences.

3. Helena Bonham Carter quoted by Krissi Murison in 'Talking Toyboys And Tiaras With The Crown's Princess Margaret', *The Times* (2 Nov. 2019). Available at: www.thetimes.co.uk/article/helena-bonham-carter-interview-talking-toyboys-and-tiaras-with-the-crowns-princess-margaret-xzqh9fcq9

4. June Jordan, 'Poem for South African Women', in *Directed by Desire: The Complete Poems of June Jordan* (Port Townsend WA: Copper Canyon Press, 2005), 278

1. THE LIFE SEASONS

1. Thinking about the business of womanhood in a Seasonal way by dividing the menstrual cycle into the four Seasons was an original concept created by Alexandra Pope and Sjanie Hugo Wurlitzer of Red School. They also developed the concepts of the Seasonal gifts and developmental tasks.

2. D. G. Blanchflower, A. J. Oswald, 'Is well-being U-shaped over the life cycle?', *Social Science & Medicine*, 66: 8 (2008), 1733–49, ISSN 0277-9536. Available at: https:/doi.org/10.1016/j.socscimed.2008.01.030.

3. A. A. Stone, J. E. Schwartz, J. E. Broderick, A. Deaton, 'A snapshot of the age distribution of psychological well-being in the United States', *Proc Natl Acad*

Sci USA., 1: 107(22) (Jun. 2010), 9985–90. DOI: 10.1073/pnas.1003744107. (Epub 17 May, 2010) PMID: 20479218; PMCID: PMC2890490. Available at: https://pubmed.ncbi.nlm.nih.gov/20479218/

3. IT'S YOUR HORMONES

1. Liz Koch, *Stalking The Wild Psoas* (Berkeley, CA: North Atlantic Books, 2019), 5.

2. For an alternative view, it's worth looking at Anthony William's work. He believes that often the problems we ascribe to menopause or thyroid issues are due to either toxicity from the environment or Epstein Barr virus (glandular fever) held in our systems. His books are listed in the resource section and many people swear by his advice. A good place to start is his book *Medical Medium* (London: Hay House, 2015).

3. Christiane Northrup, 'The multiple roles of your "reproductive" hormones', *The Wisdom of Menopause* (New York: Bantam, 2012), 48–53.

4. N. H. Bjarnason, P. Ravn, et al., 'Low body mass index is an important risk factor for low bone mass and increased bone loss in early postmenopausal women', Early Postmenopausal Intervention Cohort (EPIC) study group, *J Bone Miner Res.*, 14: 9, (1999), 1622–27. DOI: 10.1359/jbmr.1999.14.9.1622. Available at: www.ncbi.nlm.nih.gov/pubmed/10469292

5. M. Akin, 'Continuous, low-level, topical heat wrap therapy as compared to acetaminophen for primary dysmenorrhea', *J Reprod Med.* 49:9 (2004), 739–745. Available at: www.ncbi.nlm.nih.gov/pubmed/15493566

4. A HORRIBLE HISTORY OF MENOPAUSE

1. For more on this topic, check out Caroline Criado Perez's book *Invisible Women: Exposing Data Bias In A World Designed For Men* – it's fascinating stuff. How much material have you come across about the improvement in postmenopausal mental health, for example? There is still a great deal to understand about postmenopausal wellbeing which is ripe to be researched and written about by our daughters.

2. Louise Foxcroft, *Hot Flushes, Cold Science: A History of the Modern Menopause* (London: Granta Books, 2010). Kindle version, Chapter 4, 'On the borderland of pathology' and Chapter 5, 'Knives and asylums,' *loc 1987 – 3321.*

3. Robert A. Wilson, *Feminine Forever* (London: W. H. Allen, 1996).

4. W. Bazell, 'The cruel irony of trying to be "feminine forever"' (1 February, 2007). Available at:

www.nbcnews.com/id/16397237/ns/health-second_opinion/t/cruel-irony-trying-be-feminine-forever/#.XpszvVNKijg

5. Sharon Mascall, 'Time for a rethink on the clitoris', (11 June 2006). Available at: http://news.bbc.co.uk/1/hi/5013866.stm

6. Anna Moore, 'Why does medicine treat women like men?', *The Observer*, (24 May 2020). Available at: https://www.theguardian.com/society/2020/may/24/why-does-medicine-treat-women-like-men

5. MENOPAUSE GIVES US AN EVOLUTIONARY EDGE

1. 'New Evidence of Menopause in Killer Whales', *University of Exeter*, (13 July 2021). Available at: https://www.exeter.ac.uk/news/homepage/title_867602_en.html

2. Ed Yong, 'Why killer whales go through menopause but elephants don't' (5 March 2015). Available at: https://www.nationalgeographic.com/science/article/why-killer-whales-go-through-menopause-but-elephants-dont

3. Ed Yong, 'Suicidal Menopausal Aphids Save Their Colony By Sticking Themselves To Predators', (17 June 2010). Available at: https://www.nationalgeographic.com/science/article/suicidal-menopausal-aphids-save-their-colony-by-sticking-themselves-to-predators

6. YOU CAN PREPARE FOR THE PERIMENOPAUSE

1. Caitlin Moran, 'Caitlin Moran: me, drugs and the perimenopause', *The Times* (4 July, 2020).

8. SUICIDE

1. Centers For Disease Control and Prevention Available at: https://www.cdc.gov/women/lcod/2017/all-races-origins/index.htm

2. Alana Kirk, 'Why are the "sandwich generation" breaking down?', *Daily Mail* (6 July 2017). Available at: www.dailymail.co.uk/femail/article-4669026/Why-don-t-admit-t-cope-s-late.html

3. K. E. Saunders, K. Hawton, 'Suicidal behaviour and the menstrual cycle', *Psychol Med.*, 36:7 (July, 2006), 901–12. DOI: 10.1017/S0033291706007392. Epub 2006 Mar 30. PMID: 16573848. Available at: https://pubmed.ncbi.nlm.nih.gov/16573848/

If you feel suicidal

1. Brådvik L. (2018). 'Suicide Risk and Mental Disorders. *International journal of environmental research and public health'*, *15*(9), 2028. https://doi.org/10.3390/ijerph15092028

9. SYMPTOMS VARY BY CULTURE

1. Adriana Velez, 'Menopause Is Different For Women Of Color', October 2021. Available at: https://www.endocrineweb.com/menopause-different-women-color

2. Gibson, C. J., Huang, A. J., McCaw, B., Subak, L. L., Thom, D. H., & Van Den Eeden, S. K. (2019). 'Associations of Intimate Partner Violence, Sexual Assault, and Posttraumatic Stress Disorder With Menopause Symptoms Among Midlife and Older Women'. *JAMA Internal Medicine*, *179*(1), 80–87. https://doi.org/10.1001/jamainternmed.2018.5233

3. 'Team MM', 'How The Menopause Is Viewed In BAME Communities, How The Menopause Is Viewed In BAME Communities' (23 Aug. 2019), Megs Menopause, Available at: https://megsmenopause.com/2019/08/23/how-the-menopause-is-viewed-in-bame-communities-dr-nighat-arif-gp-wsi-in-women-health/

4. Ibid.

5. Amanda Randone, 'Black, Menopausal, And Opinionated: How Podcast Host Karen Arthur Found Her Voice', *Vogue* (5 Dec. 2020). Available at: www.vogue.co.uk/beauty/article/karen-arthur-interview

6. Paula Akpan, 'Why research and conversation about menopause is letting down Black and Asian people', *Good Housekeeping* (16 Feb. 2021). Available at: www.goodhousekeeping.com/uk/health/a35000306/menopause-research-healthcare-letting-down-black-and-asian-people/

7. Ibid.

8. M. Melby, 'Chilliness: A vasomotor symptom in Japan', *Menopause*, 14: 4 (2007), 752–759.

9. M. Melby, et al., 'Culture and symptom reporting at menopause', *Human Reproduction Update*, 11: 5 (2005), 495–512.

10. M. Melby, 'Vasomotor symptom prevalence and language of menopause in Japan', *Menopause*, 12: 3 (2005), 250–257.

11. Geneva Foundation for Medical Education and Research, 'Country specific information on the menopause in Japan', GMFMER (25 Oct. 2019). Available at: www.gfmer.ch/Books/bookmp/185.htm

12. Center for the Advancement of Health, 'Menopause affects Japanese women less than Westerners', *Science Daily* (27 Jul. 1998). Available at: www.science-daily.com/releases/1998/07/980727080103.htm

13. M. Martin, et al. 'Menopause without symptoms: The endocrinology of menopause among rural Mayan Indians', *Am. J. Obstet. Gyn.*, 168: 6 (1993), 1839–1843.

14. D. Stewart, 'Menopause in highland Guatemala Mayan women,' *Maturitas*, 44: 4 (2003), 293–297.

15. J. Michel, et al. Symptoms, attitudes and treatment choices surrounding menopause among the Maya of Livingston, Guatemala. *Soc. Sci. Med.*, 63: 3 (2006), 732–742.

16. K. Hawkes, 'Grandmothers and the evolution of human longevity', *Am. J. Hum. Biol.*, 15: 3 (2003), 380–400.

17. K. Hawkes, et al., 'Grandmothering, menopause, and the evolution of human life histories', *Proc. Nat. Acad. Sci.*, 95 (1998), 1–4.

18. K. Hawkes, K., et al., 'Hadza women's time allocation, offspring provisioning, and the evolution of long postmenopausal life spans', *Current Anthropology*, 38: 4 (1997), 551–577.

19. Jane Feinmann, 'As a new international study draws a surprising conclusion, we ask ... What makes British women have the worst menopause?', *Daily Mail* (15 Jun. 2010). Available at: www.dailymail.co.uk/health/article-1286569/British-women-worst-menopause.html

20. B. Ayers, M. Forshaw, and M. Hunter, 'The impact of attitudes towards the menopause on women's symptom experience: A systematic review', *Maturitas*. 65: 1 (2009). Available at: www.sciencedirect.com/science/article/abs/pii/S0378512209003971

21. K. A. Matthews, 'Myths and realities of the menopause', *Psychosom Med.*, 54: 1 (Jan-Feb., 1992), 1–9. DOI: 10.1097/00006842-199201000-00001. PMID: 1553395. Available at: https://pubmed.ncbi.nlm.nih.gov/1553395/

Self-Care Abdominal Massage

1. To learn more about Rosita Arvigo and the origins of self-care abdominal massage, see her biography *Sastun, My Apprenticeship With A Maya Healer*, published by HarperOne (1995).

10. WHEN TO USE HRT

1. NICE: National Institute for Health and Care Excellence, *Menopause: diagnosis and treatment* (5, Dec. 2019). Available at: www.nice.org.uk/guidance/ng23/chapter/Recommendations#managing-short-term-menopausal-symptoms

2. International Osteoporosis Foundation, 'Hormone replacement therapy (HRT)', osteoporosis.foundation, www.iofbonehealth.org/hormone-replacement-therapy-hrt

3. NHS, 'Could HRT stop dementia?' NHS.UK (14 Feb. 2013). Available at: www.nhs.uk/news/neurology/could-hrt-stop-dementia/

4. NHS. '"Small" increase in risk of Alzheimer's disease with HRT use, study suggests', NHS.uk. (7 Mar. 2019). Available at: www.nhs.uk/news/medication/small-increase-risk-alzheimers-disease-hrt-use-study-suggests/

5. Sarah Boseley, 'Breast cancer risk from using HRT is "twice what was thought"', *Guardian* (29 Aug. 2019). Available at: www.theguardian.com/science/2019/aug/29/breast-cancer-risk-from-using-hrt-is-twice-what-was-thought

6. Cancer Research UK, 'Does hormone replacement therapy increase cancer risk?', Cancer Research UK (27 Feb. 2019). Available at: www.cancerresearchuk.org/about-cancer/causes-of-cancer/hormones-and-cancer/does-hormone-replacement-therapy-increase-cancer-risk

7. British Heart Foundation, 'Should you be worried about HRT causing blood clots?' (11 January 2019). Available at: https://www.bhf.org.uk/informationsupport/heart-matters-magazine/news/behind-the-headlines/hrt-and-blood-clot-risk

8. Alley Einstein, Gina Clarke and Anna Roberts, 'Hormone Hell: The menopause made us suicidal,' *Sun* (28 Jun. 2018). Available at: www.thesun.co.uk/fabulous/6639625/menopause-suicidal-depression/

9. Dr Louise Newson, 'Taking HRT Forever', Episode 32. Available at: https://www.menopausedoctor.co.uk/podcasts/032-taking-hrt-forever-ann-newson-dr-louise-newson

10. Ibid.

11. WHAT TO ASK YOUR DOCTOR

1. Nuffield Health, 'One in four with menopause symptoms concerned about ability to cope with life', Nuffield Health.com (14 Sept. 2017). Available at: www.nuffieldhealth.com/article/one-in-four-with-menopause-symptoms-concerned-about-ability-to-cope-with-life

2. National Institute for Health and Care Excellence, 'Menopause: diagnosis and treatment', NICE (5 Dec. 2019). Available at: www.nice.org.uk/guidance/ng23/chapter/Recommendations#managing-short-term-menopausal-symptoms

3. Ibid.

12. COMPLEMENTARY ALLIES

1. Ardito, R. B., & Rabellino, D. (2011). 'Therapeutic alliance and outcome of psychotherapy: historical excursus, measurements, and prospects for research'. *Frontiers in psychology*, *2*, 270. Available at: https://doi.org/10.3389/fpsyg.2011.00270

2. Amanda M. Hall, Paulo H. Ferreira, Christopher G. Maher, Jane Latimer, Manuela L. Ferreira, 'The Influence of the Therapist-Patient Relationship on Treatment Outcome in Physical Rehabilitation: A Systematic Review', *Physical Therapy*, Volume 90, Issue 8, 1 August 2010, Pages 1099–1110. Available at: https://doi.org/10.2522/ptj.20090245

14. LEARNING TO REST

1. *The Week* staff, 'You should really take a nap this afternoon according to science' (10 January 2015). Available at: https://theweek.com/articles/445274/why-should-really-take-nap-afternoon-according-science

15. YOGA NIDRA – THE ULTIMATE REST

1. Matthew Thorpe, '12 Science-based benefits of meditation' (27 October 2020). Available at: https://www.healthline.com/nutrition/12-benefits-of-meditation#1.-Reduces-stress

2. Florence Elyzabeth Krieger, 'The science and benefits of yoga nidra' (15 March 2020). Available at: https://www.everydaydala.com/blog/the-science-benefits-of-yoga-nidra

3. There is an exhaustive index of research into Yoga Nidra at the Yoga Nidra Network site. Available at: www.yoganidranetwork.org/resources/academic-resources

16. THE MENSTRUALITY MEDICINE CIRCLE

1. The term 'menstruality' was coined by New Zealand psychotherapist Jane Catherine Severn in 2005. Jane Catherine Severn, 'What is Menstruality?', (1 May 2021). Available at: http://www.lunahouse.co.nz/conscious-menstruality

20. IT FEELS LIKE YOU'RE GOING MAD

1. Uma Dinsmore-Tuli, 'Interview with Alexandra Pope', *Red School* Facebook page (2 Oct. 2019). Available at: https://www.facebook.com/redschoolonline/videos/678353609338086

21. THERE ARE SOME SYMPTOMS NO ONE TELLS YOU ABOUT

1. NICE, 'Menopause: how common is it?' (November 2020). Available at: https://cks.nice.org.uk/topics/menopause/background-information/prevalence/

2. Kapoor E, Okuno M, Miller VM, Rocca LG, Rocca WA, Kling JM, Kuhle CL, Mara KC, Enders FT, Faubion SS. 'Association of adverse childhood experiences with menopausal symptoms: Results from the Data Registry on Experiences of Aging, Menopause and Sexuality (DREAMS)'. Maturitas. 2021 Jan;143:209-215. doi: 10.1016/j.maturitas.2020.10.006. Epub 2020 Oct 14. PMID: 33308631; PMCID: PMC7880696. Available at: https://pubmed.ncbi.nlm.nih.gov/33308631/

22. WHAT ABOUT EARLY MENOPAUSE?

1. Local Government Association, 'Menopause factfile'. Available at: https://www.local.gov.uk/our-support/workforce-and-hr-support/wellbeing/menopause/menopause-factfile#:~:text=In%20the%20UK%20the%20average,period%20leading%20up%20to%20menopause.

2. L. Cox, J. H. Liu, 'Primary ovarian insufficiency: an update', *Int J Women's Health*, 6 (20 Feb. 2014), 235–43. DOI: 10.2147/IJWH.S37636 Available at: www.ncbi.nlm.nih.gov/pmc/articles/PMC3934663/

3. NHS, 'Causes of Early Menopause', Available at: https://www.nhs.uk/conditions/early-menopause/

4. Ibid.

23. WHAT ABOUT INDUCED MENOPAUSE?

1. NHS, 'Considerations hysterectomy', (1 February 2019). Available at: https://www.nhs.uk/conditions/hysterectomy/considerations/

2. Newson Health, 'New Findings Recommend Oestrogen Therapy After Surgical Menopause', (16 June 2020). Available at: https://www.newson-health.co.uk/news/new-findings-recommend-oestrogen-therapy-after-surgical-menopause

3. Find out more at Sarah Miller's website: www.embodimentsdance.com.au/surgical-menopause-rites-of-passage

4. Quoted in Claudia Tanner, 'The menopause: "I came close to taking my own life – women need better support", *People*, (6 Sept. 2019). Available at: https://inews.co.uk/inews-lifestyle/people/the-menopause-i-came-close-to-taking-my-own-life-women-need-better-support-505967

5. See: Change.org. #MakeMenopauseMatter Available at: www.change.org/p/rt-hon-elizabeth-truss-mp-make-menopause-matter-in-healthcare-the-workplace-and-education-makemenopausematter?use_react=false

6. Melanie Rossiter, *Reclaiming Feminine Wisdom* (2018), Kindle version, Chapter 18 'Hysterectomy – huh?', para 4, loc 968.

7. See: Sarah Miller, Embodiments Dance Drum Circle, at: www.embodiments-dance.com.au/surgical-menopause-rites-of-passage

24. YOU ARE NOT ALONE

1. Hand in hand parenting can be found at: https://www.handinhandparenting.org/

26. TEENAGE KICKS

1. 'From womb to world', (18 March 2013), YouTube video added by TEDx Talks. Available at: https://www.youtube.com/watch?v=bZ6gLGCy84o

2. Diane Przybilla, 'My Menarche Ceremony', *Elephant Journal*, (10 July 2019). Available at: www.elephantjournal.com/2019/07/my-menarche-ceremony/

28. FOOD AND MOOD

1. K. Buchanan, J. Sheffield, 'Why do diets fail? An exploration of dieters' experiences using thematic analysis', *J Health Psychol.*, 22:7 (Jun. 2017), 906–15. DOI: 10.1177/1359105315618000. Epub 16 Dec. 2015. PMID: 26679713. Available at: https://pubmed.ncbi.nlm.nih.gov/26679713/

2. Clare Jasmine Beloved, 'Full Moon Belly', *Songs for a Sultry Spring* (poems from 2010–12). Available at: www.clarebeloved.com/products-1/songs-for-a-sultry-spring-digital-poetry-book

29. EAT WELL, FEEL WELL

1. Sally Duffell, *Grow Your Own HRT* (Scotland: Findhorn Press, 1998).

2. L. Dennerstein, 'Well-being, symptoms and the menopausal transition', *Maturitas*, 23: 2 (1996), 147–57. Available at: https://doi.org/10.1016/0378-5122(95)00970-1. Available at: https://pubmed.ncbi.nlm.nih.gov/8735353/

3. If you're interested in creating herbal remedies, Susun Weed's book *New Menopausal Years: Alternative Approaches for Women 30–90* (Woodstock: Ashtree Publishing, 2002) will tell you everything you need to know.

Super-food with a sting

1. Susun S. Weed *New Menopausal Years: Alternative Approaches for Women 30–90* (Woodstock: Ashtree Publishing, 2002) 241.

30. OUR CULTURE MAKES IT WORSE

1. Dikayak, 'Relationship between women's attitude towards menopause and quality of life', *Climacteric*, 15:6 (2012), 552–62. DOI:10.3109/13697137.2011.637651. Available at: www.ncbi.nlm.nih.gov/pubmed/22335298

2. Dorothy Sayers, *Clouds of Witness* (London: Gollancz, 1927). Published in 1927 – a year before women got the vote in the UK.

3. Mary Beard interviewed on *Woman's Hour*, BBC Radio 4 (17 Feb. 2021).

31. ENVIRONMENTAL DAMAGE

1. T. R. Brown, R. T. Zoeller, et al., 'Endocrine-disrupting chemicals and public health protection: a statement of principles from the endocrine society' quoted in Sally Duffell, *Grow Your Own HRT* (Scotland: Findhorn Press, 1998), 217.

2. Food Standards Agency, 'BPA in plastic' (12 Jan. 2018). Available at: www.food.gov.uk/safety-hygiene/bpa-in-plastic

3. Breast Cancer Action, 'Paraben-Free Cosmetics'. Available at: www.bcaction.org/our-take-on-breast-cancer/environment/safe-cosmetics/paraben-free-cosmetics/

4. Red & Honey, 'How to clean your whole house without nasty chemicals' (7 Jan. 2020) Available at: https://redandhoney.com/how-to-clean-your-whole-house-without-nasty-chemicals/

5. World Health Organization press release, 'Effects of human exposure to hormone-disrupting chemicals examined in landmark UN report', WHO (19 Feb. 2013). Available at: www.who.int/mediacentre/news/releases/2013/hormone_disrupting_20130219/en/

32. YOU WILL BE HOTTER

1. 'Estrogen and hot flashes: the hormonal link', *Menopause Now*, (18 June 2020). Available at: https://www.menopausenow.com/hot-flashes/articles/estrogen-and-hot-flashes-the-hormonal-link

2. Christophe André, 'Proper Breathing Brings Better Health', (15 January 2019). Available at: https://www.scientificamerican.com/article/proper-breathing-brings-better-health/

3. Huang AJ, Phillips S, Schembri M, Vittinghoff E, Grady D. 'Device-guided slow-paced respiration for menopausal hot flushes: a randomized controlled trial'. *Obstet Gynecol.* 2015;125(5):1130-1138. doi:10.1097/AOG.0000000000000821Available at: https://pubmed.ncbi.nlm.nih.gov/25932840/

4. Dr Christiane Northrup, *Goddesses Never Age: The Secret Prescription for Radiance, Vitality and Wellbeing* (London: Hay House, 2015), 10.

5. F. Farzaneh, et al., 'The effect of oral evening primrose oil on menopausal hot flashes: a randomized clinical trial', *Arch Gynecol Obstet*, 288 (2013), 1075–9. Available at: link.springer.com/article/10.1007%2Fs00404-013-2852-6

6. T. Odai, 'Severity of hot flushes is inversely associated with dietary intake of vitamin B_6 and oily fish', *Climacteric*, 22:6 (2019), 617-621, Available at: www.tandfonline.com/doi/full/10.1080/13697137.2019.1609440

33. TAME YOUR INNER CRITIC

1. Alexandra Pope and Sjanie Hugo Wurlitzer, *Wild Power* (London: Hay House, 2017).

35. YOUR BRAIN IS GROWING

1. A. Marcin, 'What causes menopause brain fog and how it's treated', *Healthline* (22 Dec. 2017). Available at: www.healthline.com/health/menopause/menopause-brain-fog#treatment

2. M. T. Weber, L. H. Rubin, P. M. Maki. 'Cognition in perimenopause: the effect of transition stage', *Menopause*, 20:5 (2013): 511–17. doi:10.1097/gme.0b013e31827655e5. Available at: www.ncbi.nlm.nih.gov/pubmed/23615642

3. Melissa Lee Phillips, 'The mind at midlife', American Psychological Association, 442:4 (Apr. 2011). Available at: www.apa.org/monitor/2011/04/mind-midlife

4. Christiane Northrup, *The Wisdom of Menopause* (New York: Bantam, 2012), 48–53.

5. Ibid. p.38.

6. Daniel Levitin, *The Changing Mind: A Neuroscientist's Guide to Ageing Well* (London: Penguin Life, 2020), 31–61.

36. YOUR SLEEP MAY SUFFER

1. Ekirch AR. 'Segmented Sleep in Preindustrial Societies', *Sleep*. 2016;39(3):715-716. Published 2016 Mar 1. doi:10.5665/sleep.5558 Available at: https://www.ncbi.nlm.nih.gov/pmc/articles/PMC4763365/#!po=4.16667

2. Nirlipta Tuli, Yoga Nidra Network. Available at: www.yoganidranetwork.org

3. Francis McCabe, 'Sleep Elusive? New Study Shows There's A Reason', (11 July 2017). Available at: https://www.unlv.edu/news/article/sleep-elusive-new-study-shows-there-s-reason

4. Samson DR, Crittenden AN, Mabulla IA, Mabulla AZ, Nunn CL. 'Hadza sleep biology: Evidence for flexible sleep-wake patterns in hunter-gatherers'. *Am J Phys Anthropol*. 2017 Mar;162(3):573-582. doi: 10.1002/ajpa.23160. Epub 2017 Jan 7. PMID: 28063234. Available at: https://pubmed.ncbi.nlm.nih.gov/28063234/

5. Stephanie Haggarty, 'The Myth of the Eight Hour Sleep', (22 February 2012). Available at: https://www.bbc.co.uk/news/magazine-16964783

6. Nick Littlehales, 'The secret power of napping', *Guardian* (23 Oct. 2016). Available at: www.theguardian.com/lifeandstyle/2016/oct/23/the-secret-of-power-napping

7. Christophe André, 'Proper Breathing Brings Better Health', (15 January 2019). Available at: https://www.scientificamerican.com/article/proper-breathing-brings-better-health/

8. James Nestor, *Breath: The New Science of a Lost Art* (Riverhead Books, 2020).

38. NO MORE BABIES

1. Quoted in Stephanie Marsh, '"The desire to have a child never goes away": how the involuntarily childless are forming a new movement', *Guardian* (2 Oct. 2017). Available at: www.theguardian.com/lifeandstyle/2017/oct/02/the-desire-to-have-a-child-never-goes-away-how-the-involuntarily-childless-are-forming-a-new-movement

39. RAGE AND GRIEF

1. G. Milller, et al., 'Ovulatory cycle effects on tip earnings by lap dancers: economic evidence for human estrus?', *Evolution and Human Behaviour*, 28: 6 (Nov. 2007). Available at: https://www.sciencedirect.com/science/article/abs/pii/S1090513807000694

2. Clare Dubois, 'Redefining She', (20 October 2019). Available at: https://www.facebook.com/treesisters/posts/2412864608761568

40. SURRENDER

1. Jalaluddin Rumi, 'The Guest House', *The Essential Rumi*, trans. Coleman Barks (London: Penguin, 1995), 109.

41. BE WITH THE UNKNOWN

1. Pema Chödrön, *When Things Fall Apart: Heart Advice for Difficult Times* (New York: Penguin Random House, 2016), 16.

44. SELF-CARE FOR SURRENDER

1. Audre Lorde, *A Burst of Light: And Other Essays* (Mineola: Dover Publications, 1988), 205.

45. HEAL THOSE WOUNDS

1. Tara Brach, *True Refuge* (London: Hay House, 2013).

2.   Tara Brach, 'Resources – RAIN: Recognize, Allow, Investigate, Nurture'. Available at: https://www.tarabrach.com/rain/

3.   Tara Brach, 'Meditation: Light RAIN in Difficult Times'. Available at: https://www.tarabrach.com/meditation-light-rain-difficult-times/

48. SEX CAN GET WORSE

1.   Sophie Fletcher, @mindful_menopause, 'I have a trophy vagina' Instagram post. Available at: https://www.instagram.com/p/CPGlD0Jpp3y/?utm_source=ig_web_copy_link

2.   Dr Heather Currie and Professor Grant Cumming, 'Vaginal atrophy - the taboo subject', *Menopause Matters*. Available at: https://www.menopausematters.co.uk/article-vaginal-atrophy.php

3.   Jane Lewis, *Me and My Menopausal Vagina* (PAL Books, 2018).

49. SEX CAN GET MUCH, MUCH BETTER

1.   Cally Beaton, 'Menopausal? Yes. But at 50 I'm hotter than I was in my 20s', *Guardian* (23 May 2019). Available at: www.theguardian.com/commentisfree/2019/may/23/menopausal-50-hotter-20s-older-woman?CMP=Share_iOSApp_Other

2.   Jane Fryer, 'Good golly Miss Molly! In an eye-popping interview, artist Molly Parkin, 82, reveals all about her life of hedonism', *Daily Mail* (12 Jan. 2015). Available at: www.dailymail.co.uk/femail/article-2906031/Good-golly-Miss-Molly-eye-popping-interview-artist-Molly-Parkin-82-reveals-life-hedonism-Faint-hearts-Prince-Charles-look-away-now.html

3.   K. Hutchinson, *The Last Bohemians Podcast.* (4 March 2019). Produced by Alannah Chance. Available at: https://www.thelastbohemians.co.uk/molly

4.   Quoted in *The Menopause Monologues 2*, ed. Harriet Powell (UK: Little Taboo Press, 2020), 104.

5.   Ruth Spencer, 'Libidos, vibrators and men: this is what your ageing sex drive looks like', *Guardian* (25 Mar. 2014). Available at: https://www.theguardian.com/commentisfree/2014/mar/25/aging-female-sex-drive-looks-like

50. CONTRACEPTION

1.   Katrine Bussey, 'Abortions for over-40s at record high', *The Times* (26 Aug. 2020). Available at: www.thetimes.co.uk/article/abortions-for-over-40s-at-record-high-zs96rnfwt

2. Sarah Zagorski, 'Why Are Women Over 40 Having More Abortions Than Ever Before?', LifeNews.com (13 Aug. 2014). Available at: www.lifenews.com/2014/08/13/why-are-women-over-40-having-more-abortions-than-ever-before/

3. Meg's Menopause and Dr Shahzadi Harper, *Coffee and a chat*, on Instagram 7th July 2021. Available at: https://www.instagram.com/tv/CCVV8AhBuH6/

4. The 'safely' app holds and manages information about sexual health. Available at: https://safely.me/

5. Jane Bennett and Alexandra Pope, *The Pill: Are You Sure It's for You?* (London: Allen and Unwin, 2008), 20.

6. S. A. Robinson, M. Dowell, D. Pedulla and L. McCauley, 'Do the emotional side-effects of hormonal contraceptives come from pharmacologic or psychological mechanisms?', *Med Hypotheses*. 63: 2 (2004), 268–73. Available at doi: 10.1016/j.mehy.2004.02.013. PMID: 15236788.

7. Ian Sample, 'Taking the pill could reduce women's libido, US scientists claim', *Guardian* (26 May 2005). Available at: www.theguardian.com/world/2005/may/26/research.sciencenews

8. Charlotte Wessel Skovlund, Lina Steinrud Mørch, et al., 'Association of Hormonal Contraception with Suicide Attempts and Suicides', *American Journal of Psychiatry* (17 Nov. 2017). Available at: https://doi.org/10.1176/appi.ajp.2017.17060616

9. Charlotte Wessel Skovlund, Lina Steinrud Mørch, et al., 'Association of hormonal contraception with depression', *JAMA Psychiatry*. (28 Sept. 2016). Available at: https://jamanetwork.com/journals/jamapsychiatry/fullarticle/2552796

10. Valerie Warner Findlay, Dr Katie Boog, 'Contraception for women aged over 40. What, when and for how long?' January 2018. Available at: https://www.guidelinesinpractice.co.uk/womens-health/contraception-for-women-aged-over-40-what-when-and-for-how-long/453901.article

11. L. K. Massey, M. A. Davison, 'Effects of oral contraceptives on nutritional status', *Am Fam Physician*., 19:1 (Jan. 1979), 119–23. PMID: 760421. Available at: https://pubmed.ncbi.nlm.nih.gov/760421/

12. M. Palmery, A. Saraceno, A. Vaiarelli, G. Carlomagno, 'Oral contraceptives and changes in nutritional requirements', *Eur Rev Med Pharmacol Sci*., 17: 13 (2013),1804–13. Available at: https://pubmed.ncbi.nlm.nih.gov/23852908/

13. G. E. Stark, 'Hormonal Birth Control Depletes Body of Key Nutrients', *Natural Womanhood* (6 Jan. 2021). Available at: https://naturalwomanhood.

org/is-oral-contraceptive-pill-safe-depletes-nutrients-depression-bad-for-you-092018/

14. H. Khalili, 'Risk of Inflammatory Bowel Disease with Oral Contraceptives and Menopausal Hormone Therapy: Current Evidence and Future Directions,' *Drug Saf.* 3:3 (Mar. 2016), 193–7. Doi: 10.1007/s40264-015-0372-y. PMID: 26658991; PMCID: PMC4752384. Available at: https://pubmed.ncbi.nlm.nih.gov/26658991/

15. D. Dovey, 'Birth Control Pill May Triple Risk of Crohn's Disease in Women with Family History of the Condition', *Medical Daily* (16 Mar. 2015). Available at: www.medicaldaily.com/birth-control-pill-may-triple-risk-crohns-disease-women-family-history-condition-325850

51. LUNAR CHARTING

1. Jane Bennet and Francesca Naish, *Lunar Fertility*, free eBook available at: https://www.fertility.com.au/resources/product/lunar-fertility-2/

2. Awen Clement, *Moon Wise: How to Find Peace and Power with the Cycle of the Moon* (Awen Clement, 2019).

53. YOU NEED YOUR GIRLFRIENDS

1. Mindwise Innovations, 'How friendship affects your physical and mental health', Mindwise. Available at: www.mindwise.org/blog/mental-health/how-friendship-affects-your-physical-mental-health/

2. Sarah McKay, 'Why friendship is great for your brain: a neuroscientist explains', MBG Relationships (11 Mar. 2014). Available at: www.mindbody-green.com/0-12905/why-friendship-is-great-for-your-brain-a-neuroscientist-explains.html

3. Luisa Dillner, 'Is having no social life as bad for you as smoking?', *Guardian* (11 Jan. 2016). Available at: www.theguardian.com/lifeandstyle/2016/jan/11/is-having-no-social-life-as-bad-for-you-as-smoking

4. S. L. Follis, et al., 'Psychosocial stress and bone loss among postmenopausal women: results from the Women's Health Initiative', *J Epidemiol Community Health*, 73 (2019), 888-92. Available at: https://jech.bmj.com/content/73/9/888

54. LOVE YOUR BONES

1. NHS, 'Overview: Osteoporosis' (18 Jun. 2019). Available at: www.nhs.uk/live-well/healthy-body/menopause-and-your-bone-health/

2. Columbia University Irving Medical Centre, 'Bone, not adrenaline, drives fight or flight response', *Phsy.Org* (19 Sept. 2019). Available at: https://phys. org/news/2019-09-bone-adrenaline-flight-response.html

3. G. Brunetti, et al., 'The Interplay between the bone and the immune system', *Clinical & developmental immunology* (2013), 720504. DOI: 10.1155/2013/720504 Abstract available at: www.ncbi.nlm.nih.gov/pmc/ articles/PMC3725924/

4. Paul Gallagher, 'Women over 55 going through divorce "more likely to suffer fractures due to bone loss"', The i (9 Jul. 2019). Available at: https:// inews.co.uk/news/health/post-menopausal-women-divorce-fractures-bone-loss-312022

5. H. Kumano, 'Osteoporosis and stress', *Clin Calcium.*, 15: 9 (2005), 1544–1547. See abstract at: https://www.ncbi.nlm.nih.gov/pubmed/16137956

6. Lani Simpson, *Dr. Lani's No-Nonsense Bone Health Guide* (Nashville: Hunter House, 2014).

7. A. R. Hong and S. W. Kim, 'Effects of Resistance Exercise on Bone Health', *Endocrinology and metabolism (Seoul, Korea)*, 33(4) (2018), 435–44. Available at: https://doi.org/10.3803/EnM.2018.33.4.435. See abstract at: www.ncbi.nlm.nih.gov/pmc/articles/PMC6279907/

8. G. Chang, et al., (2016). 'Twelve-Minute Daily Yoga Regimen Reverses Osteoporotic Bone Loss', *Topics in geriatric rehabilitation*, 32:2 (2016), 81–87. Available at: https://doi.org/10.1097/TGR.000000000000085. See abstract at: www.ncbi.nlm.nih.gov/pmc/articles/PMC4851231/

9. Reinagel, M. 2017 March 15th. 'Can prunes reverse bone loss?' https:// www.scientificamerican.com/article/can-prunes-reverse-bone-loss/

10. S. Hooshmand and B. H. Arjmandi, 'Viewpoint: dried plum, an emerging functional food that may effectively improve bone health', *Ageing Res Rev.*, 8:2 (2009), 122–7. DOI: 1 0.1016/j.arr.2009.01.002. See abstract at: www. ncbi.nlm.nih.gov/pubmed/19274852

11. H. M. Ochs-Balcom, et al., 'Short Sleep Is Associated With Low Bone Mineral Density and Osteoporosis in the Women's Health Initiative', *J Bone Miner Res*, 35 (2020), 261–8. DOI: 10.1002/jbmr.3879

55. THE WOMB SPEAKS

1. Hilary Lewin, 'Menopause and mining your own diamond', *Advantages of Age*. Available at: https://advantagesofage.com/exclusives/menopause-and-mining-your-diamond/

2. Tami Lynn Kent, *Wild Feminine: Finding Power, Spirit & Joy in the Female Body* (Oregon: Beyond Words), xvii.

56. YOUR 'DOWNSTAIRS' DEPARTMENT SPEAKS

1. Rosa Farah and Anita J. Ribeiro, 'Excerpts from Jung's Work Related to Body and Psyche', *Calatonia*. Available at: www.calatonia.org/en/excerpts-from-jungs-work-related-to-body-and-psyche-compiled-by-rosa-farah-anita-j-ribeiro/

2. Excerpt from 'Ask Your Body' reproduced with the kind permission of Kai Siedenburg from her collection *Poems of Earth and Spirit* (Santa Cruz: Our Nature Connection, 2017), 59.

57. WE NEED A GAP YEAR

1. K. Pickering, J. Bennett, *About Bloody Time* (Melbourne: Victorian Women's Trust, 2019), 31.

2. Frances Lewis, interviewed about her menopause gap on Stories of the Journey Home podcast: '*The Journey of Menopause with Frances Lewis*'. Available at: https://storiesofthejourneyhome.com/the-journey-of-menopause-with-frances-lewis/

3. Adelina Abad-Pedrosa and Frances Lewis, *The Divine Dance in the Sacred Landscape of Britain* (Ohio: In The Garden Publishing, 2012).

58. MENOPAUSE AT WORK

1. Rebecca Lewis and Louise Newson, 'Menopause at Work: a survey to look at the impact of menopausal and perimenopausal symptoms upon women in the workplace' (4 Jul. 2019). Available at: https://d2931px9t312xa.cloudfront.net/menopausedoctor/files/information/323/Lewis%20%20Newson%20BMS%20poster%20SCREEN%20(1).pdf

2. BMA. 'Challenging the culture on menopause for working doctors' (2020). Available at: www.bma.org.uk/media/2913/bma-challenging-the-culture-on-menopause-for-working-doctors-report-aug-2020.pdf

3. Sally Leach, 'Menopause tribunals: what can employers learn?' (16 July 2018).

Available at: https://menopauseintheworkplace.co.uk/employment-law/tribunals-employers-best-practice/

4. Unison. *The Menopause is a Workplace Issue: Guidance and Model Policy* (London: Unison). Brochure available at: www.unison.org.uk/content/uploads/2019/10/25831.pdf

5. Government Equalities Office, 'Think, act, report: Marks and Spencer' (7 October 2013). Available at: https://www.gov.uk/government/case-studies/marks-spencer-recruiting-women-from-different-backgrounds

6. S. Boseley, H. Osborne, 'Workplaces must protect women going through menopause, say MPs', *Guardian* (25 Aug. 2019). Available at: www.theguardian.com/society/2019/aug/25/mandatory-workplace-menopause-policies-uk

7. Employee Rescue, 'Menopause problems at work' (1 March 2020). Available at: www.employeerescue.co.uk/advice/problems-at-work/dealing-with-menopause-problems-at-work/

60. YOU WILL BE ASKED TO LET GO SOME MORE

1. Brené Brown, '*The Midlife Unravelling*' (24 Mar. 2018). Available at: https://brenebrown.com/blog/2018/05/24/the-midlife-unraveling/

62. LEARNING TO TRUST

1. Melanie Santorini, *Majesteria: Spiritual Guidance: Through the Menopausal Gateway* (USA: Balboa Press, 2019), Kindle version, Chapter 9, 'Retreating into the depths', paragraph 3, loc 1335.

63. HOLDING THE CHARGE

1. Alexandra Pope and Sjanie Hugo Wurlitzer, *Wild Power* (London: Hay House), 85.

65. FINDING YOUR CALLING

1. Annie Dillard, *The Writing Life* (New York: Harper Perennial, 1990), 32.

66. MAKE FRIENDS WITH DEATH

1. Stephen Levine, *A Year to Live: How to Live This Year as If It Were Your Last* (Boston: Beacon Press, 1997).

2. Z. Schachter-Shalomi, *From Age-ing to Sage-ing: A Revolutionary Approach to Growing Older* (New York: Grand Central Publishing, 1997).

67. REDEFINE HOW TO BE A WOMAN

1. AARP Research, 'The magazine study on divorce finds that women are doing the walking but both sexes are reaping rewards in the bedroom', AARP.org. (May 2004). Available at: www.aarp.org/research/topics/life/info-2014/divorce.html

2. Darcey Steinke, *Flash Count Diary: A New Story About Menopause* (Edinburgh: Canongate, 2020), Kindle edition, Chapter 5, 'Demigirl in Kemmering', para 9, loc 913.

3. M. Pekker, 'Why some women change sexual identity in midlife', *Menopause-aid* (3 Feb. 2013). Available at: https://menopause-aid.blogspot.com/2013/02/why-some-women-change-sexual-identity.html

4. Hélène Tragos Stelian, '8 things later-in-life lesbians want you to know', (6 December 2017), *HuffPost*. Available at: www.huffpost.com/entry/things-lesbians-want-you-to-know_b_8577926

68. WE NEED ROLE MODELS

1. Penny's website is https://www.pennysimkin.com/

2. *Fleabag*, Season Two, episode 3, directed by Harry Bradbeer, written by Phoebe Waller-Bridge.

3. *Herstory Movie, The Visionary Life of Lydia Ruyle and the Banners of the Divine Feminine*, directed by Dr Isadora, 2019 theherstorymovie.com

4. Philip Pullman, *The Book of Dust: Volume Two, The Secret Commonwealth* (London: Penguin and David Fickling Books, 2019), 306.

5. Viv Albertine, *To Throw Away Unopened* (London: Faber & Faber, 2018) Chapter 11 'I turn away from the smokers, Fishwife', para 10, loc 656.

6. Viv Albertine, 'Confessions of a MILF', from the album *The Vermillion Border* (Universal, 2013). Song available at: https://www.youtube.com/watch?v=RdBeYG4Ct7E

69. YOU WILL ENTER SECOND SPRING

1. A. Campbell, P. Stockley, 'Female competition and aggression: interdisciplinary perspectives', *Phil. Trans. R. Soc.* 368: 1631 (5 Dec. 2013). Available at: http://doi.org/10.1098/rstb.2013.0073

2. J. Y. Zhuang, J. X. Wang, 'Women ornament themselves for intrasexual competition near ovulation, but for intersexual attraction in luteal phase', *PLoS One*, 9: 9 (2. Sep. 2014). Available at: doi:10.1371/journal.pone.0106407.

3. *Menopause and Me* (BBC, 2017), presented by Kirsty Wark, produced by Shiona McCubbin.

4. Jean Shinoda Bolen, *Crones Don't Whine: Concentrated Wisdom for Juicy Women* (Newburyport, Mass.: Conari Press, 2003), 3.

Resources

AUDIO PRACTICES TO DOWNLOAD

Available for you at katecodrington.co.uk/second-spring-downloads/
- Clearing Meditation
- Circle
- Womb Journey Meditation
- Yoga Nidra for Separation
- Yoga Nidra for Surrender
- Yoga Nidra for Emergence
- Yoga Nidra for Second Spring
- Menstrual and moon charts

BOOKS I LOVE

AGEING WELL

Stephen Levine, *A Year to Live: How to Live This Year as If It Were Your Last* (Boston: Beacon Press, 1997).

Zalman Schachter-Shalomi, *From Age-ing To Sage-ing: A Revolutionary Approach To Growing Older* (New York: Grand Central Publishing, 1997).

BREATHING

James Nestor, *Breath: A New Science of a Lost Art* (New York: Riverhead Books, 2020).

CONTRACEPTION

Jane Bennett and Alexandra Pope, *The Pill: Are You Sure It's for You?* (London: Allen and Unwin, 2008).

Jane Bennet and Francesca Naish, *Lunar Fertility* (free eBook from fertility.com. au).

FOOD

Sally J. Duffell, *Grow Your Own HRT* (Scotland: Findhorn Press, 1998).

Giulia Enders, *Gut* (London: Scribe UK, 2017).

Susie Orbach, *On Eating: Change Your Eating, Change Your Life* (London: Penguin, 2002).

Anthony William, *Medical Medium: Secrets Behind Chronic and Mystery Illness and How to Finally Heal* (London: Hay House, 2015).

HISTORY

Louise Foxcroft, *Hot Flushes, Cold Science: A History of the Modern Menopause* (London: Granta, 2010).

Gabrielle Jackson, *Pain and Prejudice: A Call to Arms for Women and their Bodies* (London: Piatkus, 2019).

MEMOIR, FICTION, AND PERSONAL STORIES

Viv Albertine, *Clothes, Clothes, Clothes. Music, Music, Music. Boys, Boys, Boys* (London: Faber & Faber, 2015).

Viv Albertine, *To Throw Away Unopened* (London: Faber & Faber, 2019).

Jane Cawthorne and E. D. Morin eds., *Writing Menopause: An Anthology of Fiction, Poetry and Creative Non-Fiction* (Toronto: Ianna Publications, 2017).

Katrina Kenison. *Magical Journey: An Apprenticeship in Contentment* (New York: Grand Central Publishing, 2013).

Melanie Rossiter, *Reclaiming Feminine Wisdom: An Empowering Journey With Endometriosis* (independently published, 2018).

Melonie Santorini, *Majesteria: Spiritual Guidance: Through the Menopausal Gateway* (USA: Balboa Press, 2019).

The Menopause Monologues 1 and 2, compiled and edited by Harriet Powell (UK: Little Taboo Press, 2019 and 2020).

Darcey Steinke, *Flash Count Diary: A New Story About Menopause* (Edinburgh: Canongate, 2020).

Tara Westover, *Educated* (London: Windmill Books, 2018).

MENSTRUATION

Claire Baker, *50 Things You Should Know About Periods: Know Your Flow and Live in Sync with your Cycle* (London: Pavilion, 2020).

Lara Briden, *Period Repair Manual, Natural Treatment for Better Hormones and Better Periods* (Lara Briden, 2017).

Maisie Hill, *Period Power: Harness Your Hormones and Get Your Cycle Working For You* (Green Tree, 2019).

Lisa Lister *Code Red, Know Your Flow, Unlock Your Superpowers, and Create a Bloody Amazing Life. Period.* (London: Hay House, 2020).

Karen Pickering and Jane Bennett, *About Bloody Time* (Melbourne: Victorian Women's Trust, 2019).

Alexandra Pope and Sjanie Hugo Wurlitzer *Wild Power: Discover the Magic of Your Menstrual Cycle and Awaken the Feminine Path to Power* (London: Hay House, 2017).

MINDFULNESS

Tara Brach, *True Refuge: Finding Peace And Freedom in Your Own Awakened Heart* (London: Hay House, 2013).

Kim Davies, *Practical Mindfulness: Simple Techniques to Become Calmer, Happier and More Focused in Daily Life* (London: Lorenz Books, 2017).

Sophie Fletcher, *Mindful Menopause, How to Have a Calm and Positive Menopause* (London:Vermillion, 2021).

POETRY

Clare Jasmine Beloved, *Songs for a Sultry Spring*, available at: www.clarebeloved.com/products-1/songs-for-a-sultry-spring-digital-poetry-book

Kai Siedenburg, *Poems of Earth and Spirit* (Santa Cruz: Our Nature Connection, 2017).

PRACTICAL

Awen Clement, *Moon Wise* (Awen Clement, 2019).

Uma Dinsmore-Tuli, *Yoni Shakti* (YogaWords, 2020).

Sara Gottfried, *The Hormone Cure: Reclaim Balance, Sleep and Sex Drive; Lose Weight; Feel Focused, Vital, and Energized Naturally with the Gottfried Protocol* (New York: Simon & Schuster, 2014).

Tami Lynn Kent, *Wild Feminine: Finding Power, Spirit & Joy in the Female Body* (London: Atria, 2011).

Jane Lewis, *Me and My Menopausal Vagina* (PAL Books, 2018).

Christiane Northrup, *The Wisdom of Menopause: Creating Physical and Emotional Health During the Change* (New York: Bantam, 2012).

— *Goddesses Never Age: The Secret Prescription for Radiance, Vitality and Wellbeing* (London: Hay House, 2015).

Kathryn Petras, *Premature Menopause Book* (New York: William Morrow, 2018).

Marcelle Pick, *Is It Me Or My Hormones?: The Good, the Bad, and the Ugly about PMS, Perimenopause, and All the Crazy Things That Occur with Hormone Imbalance* (London: Hay House, 2013).

Lani Simpson, *Dr Lani's No-Nonsense Bone Health Guide: The Truth about Density Testing, Osteoporosis Drugs and Building Bone Quality at Any Age* (Nashville: Hunter House, 2014).

Susun Weed, *New Menopausal Years: Alternative Approaches for Women 30–90* (Woodstock: Ashtree Publishing, 2002).

SOULFUL

Suzanne Braun Levine, *The Woman's Guide to Second Adulthood: Inventing the Rest of Our Lives* (London: Bloomsbury, 2005).

— *You Gotta Have Girlfriends: A Post-Fifty Posse Is Good for Your Health* (Open Road Media, 2013).

Bonnie J. Horrigan, *Red Moon Passage* (Harmony Books, 1996).

Frances Lewis and Adelina Abad-Pedrosa, *The Divine Dance in the Sacred Landscape of Britain* (Ohio: In The Garden Publishing, 2012).

Clarissa Pinkola Estes, *Women Who Run With The Wolves* (London: Rider Books, 2008).

Joan Shinoda Bolen, *Crones Don't Whine: Concentrated Wisdom for Juicy Women* (Newburyport, Mass.: Conari Press, 2003).

TRAUMA

Richard Grannon, *How To Stop An Emotional Flashback* (Kindle, 2016).

Peter Levine, *Waking the Tiger: Healing Trauma* (Berkeley, CA: North Atlantic Books, 1997).

Arielle Schwartz, *Complex PTSD Workbook* (USA: PESI Publishing Inc, 2021).

Jasmin Lee Cori, *Healing From Trauma* (USA: Da Capo Lifelong Books, 2009).

WEBSITES I LOVE

BLACK MENOPAUSE

Black Girls' Guide to Surviving Menopause: https://blackgirlsguidetosurvivingmenopause.com/

Menopause Whilst Black podcast: https://podcasts.apple.com/gb/podcast/menopause-whilst-black/id1537012198

@MenopauseWhilstBlack for Karen Arthur's Instagram.

CHILD-FREE AND CHILDLESS RESOURCES

childlessbychoiceproject.com for those who have chosen not to have children.
fertilitynetworkuk.org for information on fertility.
gateway-women.com for support and inspiration for childless women.
saltwaterandhoney.org for stories about infertility, childlessness and faith.

COMMUNITIES

Search in Facebook for *The Menopause Support Network* for #MakeMenopauseMatter,
Diane Danzebrink's group.
Search in Facebook for Vaginal Atrophy to find Jane Lewis's support group (she
wrote *My Menopausal Vagina*).

CONTRACEPTION

naturalwomanhood.org for all about natural fertility methods.
nfpta.org.uk to find a natural family-planning teacher.
sexwise.org.uk for clear information about contraception.

DYING

deathcafe.com for talking about and planning for living and dying.
naturaldeath.org.uk is the home of the Natural Death Society, a great place to
learn about dying.

EARLY MENOPAUSE AND HYSTERECTOMY

daisynetwork.org.uk for information and support for early menopause.
earlymenopause.com for help and resources for early and for surgical menopause.
hystersisters.com is a fantastic support option for those who've entered early
menopause due to hysterectomy.

GYNAE HEALTH

Eveappeal.org.uk/nurse or freephone 0808 802 0019 or email nurse@eveappeal.
org.uk free, specialist gynaecological information service.

HEALTH RESOURCES

dutchtest.com to order your DUTCH (dried urine test for comprehensive hormones) test.
livestrong.com/article/215001-what-is-a-dim-supplement information on DIM
supplements which contain diindolylmethane, a component of cruciferous veggies.
menopausedoctor.co.uk for clear information and up-to-date research on hormone
therapy.

nice.org.uk for National Institute for Health and Care Excellence (aka NICE) treatment guidelines for HRT and all other health condition in UK.

PRODUCTS
clarebeloved.com for beautiful clothes, artwork, and courses with Clare Jasmine Beloved.
intothewylde.com for *Into The Wylde* herb and water-based organic lube.
yesyesyes.org for *YES*, water-based and oil based, organic lube.
sh-womenstore.com, a sex and pleasure shop for women.
skysprouts.co.uk to buy organic seeds for sprouting.

RAIN MEDITATION
Tarabrach.com to find more about Tara Brach's RAIN meditation.

RITUALS: PEOPLE WHO OFFER MENARCHE AND CRONING RITUALS
Angie Litvinof: angielitvinoff.com
Melonie Syrett: meloniesyrett.com.
Clare Warren: clarityvibration.com

SECOND SPRING ICONS
pinterest.co.uk/KateCodrington/second-spring-summer-inspiration for a growing portfolio of *Second Spring* icons – pop over and add your own!
theherstorymovie.com to watch the inspirational film about Lydia Rules, her glorious Second Spring and attitude towards death.

SUICIDE HELPLINES
UK
Campaign Against Living Miserably – CALM, phone: 0800 58 58 58, web: thecalmzone.net
Samaritans, phone: 116 123, web: samaritans.org

US
National Suicide Prevention Lifeline, phone: 1-800-273-8255 suicidepreventionlifeline.org
Samaritans, phone: (877) 870-4673

THERAPIES
abmt.org.uk for Biodynamic therapy and massage.
acupuncture.org.uk for acupuncture.
bacp.co.uk or psychotherapy.org.uk for counselling or psychotherapy.

csp.org.uk search here for women's health physiotherapists.
fertilitymassage.co.uk or abdominal-sacralmassage.com for abdominal massage.
ifm.org for Functional Medicine.
nimh.org.uk or bhma.info for herbalists.
redschool.net/menstrual-medicine-circle-facilitators for Menstruality Medicine
    Circle facilitators.
shiatsusociety.org for shiatsu.
WellDoing.org is a therapist matching service.
wildfeminine.com/contact/ for *Holistic Pelvic Care*® practitioners.
ukhypopressives.com to find hypopressive teachers.
Lottie Randomly, @know.your.cycle on Instagram

TRANS AND NON-BINARY
kennyethanjones.com or @kennyethanjones on Instagram.
queermenopause.com or @queermenopause on Instagram.
queersexedcc.com or @queersexedcc on Instagram.
transcare.ucsf.edu/guidelines/bone-health-and-osteoporosis for information on
    bone health.
transcare.ucsf.edu/guidelines/pain-transmen trans pelvic pain and periods.

WORKPLACE
menopauseintheworkplace.co.uk information, training and information on
    menopause policies in the workplace.
henpicked.net information and training

WORKSHOPS, ONLINE COURSES AND RETREATS
woman-kind.co.uk for online and in-person courses and retreats for menopause.
redschoolonline.net for Red School online courses on menarche and menstruation.
thewiserwoman.com/course Tania Elfersy's Wiser Woman course for natural
    symptom relief.

YOGA NIDRA
Yoganidranetwork.org for free yoga nidras of every kind.

XENOESTROGENS
breastcanceruk.org.uk has a comprehensive list of products that are paraben free.
gov.uk/safety-hygiene/bpa-in-plastic for up to date information on plastics.
redandhoney.com/how-to-clean-your-whole-house-without-nasty-chemicals/
    hormone friendly cleaning.

ONE PLACE. MANY STORIES

Bold, innovative and
empowering publishing.

FOLLOW US ON:

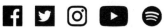

@HQStories